# The Parkinson's Plate

# The Parkinson's Plate

## A HEALTH & DIET GUIDE TO MANAGE YOUR JOURNEY

Dr. Michael S. Okun, MD
& Emily Truscott, MS, RD, LD

Robert ROSE

For complete cataloguing information, see page 256.

**Disclaimer**
This book is a general guide only and should never be a substitute for the skill, knowledge and experience of a qualified medical professional dealing with the facts, circumstances and symptoms of a particular case.

The nutritional, medical and health information presented in this book is based on the research, training and professional experience of the authors, and is true and complete to the best of their knowledge. However, this book is intended only as an informative guide for those wishing to know more about health, nutrition and medicine; it is not intended to replace or countermand the advice given by the reader's personal physician. Because each person and situation is unique, the authors and the publisher urge the reader to check with a qualified health-care professional before using any procedure where there is a question as to its appropriateness. A physician should be consulted before beginning any exercise program. The authors and the publisher are not responsible for any adverse effects or consequences resulting from the use of the information in this book. It is the responsibility of the reader to consult a physician or other qualified health-care professional regarding his or her personal care.

The recipes in this book have been carefully tested by our kitchen and our tasters. To the best of our knowledge, they are safe and nutritious for ordinary use and users. For those people with food or other allergies, or who have special food requirements or health issues, please read the suggested contents of each recipe carefully and determine whether or not they may create a problem for you. All recipes are used at the risk of the consumer.

We cannot be responsible for any hazards, loss or damage that may occur as a result of any recipe use.

For those with special needs, allergies, requirements or health problems, in the event of any doubt, please contact your medical adviser prior to the use of any recipe.

At the time of publication, all URLs linked to existing websites. Robert Rose Inc. is not responsible for maintaining, and does not endorse the content of, any website or content not created by Robert Rose Inc.

Design and Production: Kevin Cockburn/PageWave Graphics Inc.
Editor: Amy Treadwell
Proofreader: Kelly Jones
Indexer: Gillian Watts

Front cover image: © Getty Images
Illustrations: © Getty Images

Published by Robert Rose Inc.
120 Eglinton Avenue East, Suite 800, Toronto, Ontario, Canada M4P 1E2
Tel: (416) 322-6552 Fax: (416) 322-6936
www.robertrose.ca

Printed and bound in China

1 2 3 4 5 6 7 8 9 ESP 34 33 32 31 30 29 28 27 26

To all the people touched by Parkinson's,
we dedicate this book to their journey and
to their pursuit of a more meaningful life.

# CONTENTS

# PART I

# UNDERSTANDING PARKINSON'S DISEASE

CHAPTER 1

# LIVING WITH PARKINSON'S DISEASE

*At its core, Parkinson's disease reflects a problem in how certain brain cells and circuits function and survive.*

Parkinson's disease is not a single moment in time. It is a journey that unfolds slowly, often quietly, and almost always differently from one person to the next. Emily and I have spent our careers walking alongside folks living with Parkinson's disease, their families and their care partners, and if there is one truth that rises above all others, it is this: Parkinson's is more than a movement disorder, and it is more than a diagnosis. It is a whole-body condition that touches biology, behavior, emotions, relationships and daily life.

## What Is Happening in the Brain in Parkinson's?

At its core, Parkinson's disease reflects a problem in how certain brain cells and circuits function and survive. The cells most closely linked to Parkinson's produce dopamine, a chemical messenger that helps coordinate movement, motivation, learning and reward. These cells are located in a small but powerful region of the brain called the substantia nigra. As Parkinson's progresses, these dopamine-producing cells become stressed and are gradually lost. It is important to remember that Parkinson's disease is not just a disease of dopamine. There are many brain circuits and brain chemicals that are damaged and lost in the process of the degeneration.

One hallmark seen in the brains of many individuals with Parkinson's is the accumulation of a protein called alpha synuclein. Instead of folding normally and being cleared away, this protein can clump together and disrupt how brain cells work. These protein-based changes do not stay confined to one spot. Over time, they can affect interconnected brain networks that regulate movement, mood, sleep, thinking and even the gut.

It is important to emphasize that Parkinson's biology is complex. Dopamine loss matters; however, it is not the whole story. Other brain chemicals such as serotonin, norepinephrine and acetylcholine are also involved. This broader network disruption helps explain why Parkinson's includes non-movement symptoms and why treatments must go beyond simply replacing dopamine.

**RISK FACTORS**

- Parkinson's rarely has a single cause. It is usually a combination of age, genetics, and environment working together.
- Age is the strongest risk factor. As we age, the brain becomes less efficient at clearing damaged proteins.
- Genetics matter, but only a small percentage of cases are caused by a single gene change.
- Environmental exposures such as pesticides, industrial chemicals, and air pollution may increase risk.
- Early warning conditions may include REM sleep behavior disorder, constipation, and loss of smell.
- Head injury and changes in gut health are also being actively studied.
- The goal is not blame. The goal is understanding risk so that we can think about prevention and earlier detection.

## Risk Factors and Vulnerability

Most folks ask a simple and very human question: Why did this happen to me? The honest answer is that Parkinson's usually arises from a combination of vulnerabilities rather than a single cause.

Age is the strongest risk factor. As the brain ages, its ability to handle stress and clear damaged proteins is reduced. Genetics also play a role. Some individuals carry gene variants that increase risk, although for most people genetics alone are not the full explanation. Only about 13% of people with Parkinson's have a single change in their genes responsible for their Parkinson's symptoms.

Environmental exposures are increasingly recognized as contributors. Certain pesticides, industrial chemicals and air pollutants have been linked to higher Parkinson's risk. Head injury, sleep disorders such as rapid eye movement (REM) sleep behavior disorder, and changes in the gut microbiome are also being actively studied as pieces of the puzzle. What matters most is not assigning blame; however, understanding risk helps us think about prevention, earlier detection and healthier choices, especially as we move forward.

## The Parkinson's Disease Symptoms and How They Show Up

Parkinson's symptoms are frequently divided by leading experts into motor and non-motor features; however, in real life the symptoms all blend. Motor symptoms include slowness of movement, stiffness, tremor, changes in balance and alterations in walking. These symptoms can affect handwriting, facial expression, posture and the ease of everyday tasks like buttoning a shirt or rising from a chair. Non-motor symptoms in contrast are frequently just as impactful, and sometimes more so. These can include constipation, sleep disturbances, fatigue, pain, apathy, anxiety, depression, changes in thinking, and difficulties with attention or memory. Loss of smell, lightheadedness when standing, and changes in blood pressure or sweating are also common features of Parkinson's disease.

Because these symptoms may appear years before a diagnosis, many folks do not immediately connect them to Parkinson's. Over time, the accumulation of symptoms can affect independence, confidence and quality of life.

Three symptoms that commonly appear early in Parkinson's disease and may appear before motor symptoms include:

- Loss of smell
- Constipation
- Acting out of dreams (REM sleep behavior disorder)

## The Impact of Parkinson's Disease on Daily Living and on Your Health

Living with Parkinson's means constantly adapting. Your energy levels may fluctuate. Good days and harder days can occur back to back and this can trigger frustration. Planning, pacing and flexibility become essential skills for people living with Parkinson's disease.

Physical health can be influenced by changes in movement, swallowing, digestion and nutrition. Weight loss or weight gain may occur. Reduced activity can affect bone health and cardiovascular fitness, while stiffness and pain can discourage movement even though exercise is one of the most powerful tools we have to treat Parkinson's disease.

Emotional health matters deeply. Anxiety and depression are not signs of weakness. They are part of the biology of Parkinson's and deserve recognition and treatment. Social connections, purpose and joy are protective factors that should be nurtured alongside Parkinson's disease medications and therapies.

## Why Food and Lifestyle Belong in the Parkinson's Disease Conversation

Understanding Parkinson's disease provides context for every choice that follows and one of the most powerful ways to live better with Parkinson's disease is to address your diet.

### PARKINSON'S SYMPTOMS

#### MOTOR SYMPTOMS

- Slowness of movement (bradykinesia)
- Stiffness or rigidity
- Tremor (often at rest), not present in everyone
- Balance problems and falls
- Changes in walking and posture

#### NON-MOTOR SYMPTOMS

- Constipation
- Sleep problems (including acting out dreams)
- Fatigue
- Depression and anxiety
- Apathy and low motivation
- Cognitive changes (thinking, memory, attention)
- Loss of smell
- Lightheadedness or blood pressure changes
- Pain and sensory changes

Nutrition does not cure Parkinson's; however, food influences energy, digestion, medication response, inflammation and overall well-being. Meals can be a source of nourishment, pleasure and control in a condition that often feels unpredictable.

Living well with Parkinson's is about stacking small advantages. Knowledge is one. Movement is another. Sleep, stress management, social connection and thoughtful nutrition all can be woven together to support brain and body health.

As you move through this book, remember that although Parkinson's is part of your story, it does not define the whole narrative. With the right tools, the right support and the right information, many folks can and will continue to live meaningful, engaged and fulfilling lives. This chapter is the foundation. What comes next is about helping you thrive.

### LIVING WELL WITH PARKINSON'S

- Living well is about stacking small advantages every day.
- Movement, nutrition, sleep, and stress management all work together.
- Parkinson's care should be proactive, not reactive.
- You are not just treating symptoms, you are building resilience.
- Social connection and purpose are powerful forms of medicine.
- Flexibility matters. Good days and hard days will both happen.
- Parkinson's is part of your story, however it does not define your future.

## References

Bloem BR, Okun MS, Klein C. Parkinson's disease. *Lancet.* 2021 Jun 12;397(10291):2284-2303. doi: 10.1016/S0140-6736(21)00218-X. Epub 2021 Apr 10. PMID: 33848468.

Okun MS, Bloem BR, Dorsey ER. The Parkinson's Universe: A person-centered care model for Parkinson's disease. *J Parkinsons Dis.* 2026 Feb;16(1):192-195. doi: 10.1177/1877718X251399958. Epub 2025 Dec 3. PMID: 41334725.

Okun MS, Malaty IA, Deeb W. *Living with Parkinson's Disease: A Complete Guide for Patients and Caregivers.* Toronto: Robert Rose, 2020.

CHAPTER 2

# CURRENT MANAGEMENT STRATEGIES

*Nutrition, which is the focus of this book, is woven through all these strategies and interacts with nearly every treatment decision.*

Parkinson's disease is treatable. That statement matters, and it deserves to be frequently vocalized. While we do not yet have a cure, we have many effective strategies that can reduce symptoms, preserve function and improve quality of life. The challenge is not a lack of options. The challenge is knowing how to use the right tools, in the right combination, at the right time, for the right person.

Parkinson's is a long journey. Management is not a single decision or a single prescription. It is a dynamic process that evolves as your symptoms change, your life circumstances shift and the science advances. The most successful approaches recognize Parkinson's as a whole-body condition and will treat it accordingly.

This chapter lays out the core pillars of current Parkinson's management. These include medications, surgical and device-based therapies, rehabilitation strategies, mental health support, lifestyle interventions and the central role of the care team. Nutrition, which is the focus of this book, is woven through all these strategies and interacts with nearly every treatment decision.

## The Philosophy of Parkinson's Care

Before discussing specific treatments, it helps to define a guiding philosophy. Parkinson's care works best when it is proactive rather than reactive. Waiting until symptoms are severe or disabling is rarely the best approach. Instead, the goal should be to anticipate problems, adjust early and support long-term brain and body health.

Equally important is personalization. No two folks experience Parkinson's in the same way. Symptoms vary. Medication responses differ. Life goals are not identical. Effective management respects these differences and avoids a one-size-fits-all mindset.

Finally, Parkinson's care works best when folks are empowered. Understanding options, asking questions, tracking symptoms and participating in decisions all improve outcomes.

## Medications: One of the Key Foundations for Symptom Control

For most folks, medications form the backbone of Parkinson's treatment. These therapies primarily aim to restore or support dopamine signaling in the brain, although some target other chemical systems and circuits involved in movement and in non-motor symptoms.

### WHY DOPAMINE IS IMPORTANT

Dopamine is a chemical messenger that helps your brain coordinate movement, motivation, learning, and reward. In Parkinson's, the cells that make dopamine are gradually lost. When dopamine levels drop, movements become slower and less coordinated, and non-motor symptoms such as mood and motivation can also be affected. Replacing or supporting dopamine is one of the central strategies in Parkinson's treatment.

### Levodopa and carbidopa

Levodopa remains the most effective medication for treatment of Parkinson's motor symptoms. Levodopa is converted into dopamine in the brain and directly addresses the chemical deficiency driving slowness, stiffness and tremor.

Carbidopa is a drug paired with levodopa to prevent the breakdown of the medication before it reaches the brain and to reduce side effects such as nausea. Together, these medications can dramatically improve movement and function.

Despite decades of use, levodopa is often misunderstood. Levodopa does not accelerate Parkinson's progression. It does not poison the brain. When used appropriately, it improves quality of life and can reduce complications by enabling movement, exercise and independence.

The timing of your Parkinson's disease therapies matters. Levodopa works best when taken on a consistent schedule. Protein in food can interfere with absorption in some but not all folks, which is why meal timing and food choices become relevant. This interaction is not a reason to avoid protein; however, it may require some proactive planning.

### FACTS ABOUT SINEMET

- The word "*sine*" in Latin translates to "without."
- The word "*emetic*" translates to "emesis," or "causing vomiting."
- Sinemet is a combination of carbidopa/levodopa designed to treat Parkinson's disease and to block vomiting. The carbidopa blocks the vomiting.
- Carbidopa is a dopa decarboxylase inhibitor.

## HOW CAN I DECIDE ON A MEDICATION?

Choosing a medication can be tricky and stressful and should involve detailed conversations, over time, with your doctor. You and your doctor can review the different available options and assess the risks and benefits of each of these choices, but the discussion should always focus on your particular symptoms. The decision for or against a specific medication is more complex than the simple list of side effects. Your body's reaction to the medication might not match the expected benefit/risk profile for a number of reasons, including your own metabolism and any medical conditions that you have other than Parkinson's disease.

### COMMON CLASSES OF MEDICATIONS

| CLASS OF MEDICATION | EXAMPLES |
| --- | --- |
| Levodopa preparations | Carbidopa/levodopa combination (Sinemet), benserazide/levodopa (Madopar) |
| Dopamine agonists | Ropinirole, pramipexole, rotigotine |
| Monoamine oxidase type B (MAO-B) inhibitors | Selegiline, rasagiline, safinamide |
| Catechol-O-methyltransferase (COMT) inhibitors | Entacapone, tolcapone, opicapone |
| Others | Trihexyphenidyl, amantadine, istradefylline |

Finally, dopamine treatments can result in nausea. There are several approaches that can be employed to address this potential side effect, such as adding carbidopa, changing the formulation or using a medication called domperidone.

### Dopamine agonists

Dopamine agonists mimic dopamine; however, instead of simply replacing dopamine, they directly stimulate the dopamine receptors in your brain. They are often used in younger individuals or as an add-on therapy to levodopa.

These medications can reduce motor symptoms. However, this class of medications carries unique risks, including sleepiness, swelling, hallucinations and impulse control behaviors such as compulsive gambling, shopping or hypersexuality.

Careful monitoring of dopamine agonists is essential. When used thoughtfully, dopamine agonists can be helpful. When misused or poorly monitored, they can cause significant harm. The monitoring plan for dopamine agonists should always involve a spouse, family member or close friend as the person may be unaware of the impulse control symptoms.

## THINGS TO KNOW ABOUT THE USE OF DOPAMINE AGONISTS

- Experts no longer uniformly recommend that a dopamine agonist must be used before levodopa.
- Dopamine agonists can be used alone in monotherapy or in combinations with other medications.
- Dopamine agonists are longer-acting than levodopa.
- The most concerning side effect to monitor is impulse control disorder.
- Another concerning side effect is sudden sleepiness (which may affect driving).

### MAO-B inhibitors and COMT inhibitors

These two extend the effect of dopamine by slowing its breakdown in the brain or body. These medications are often used early in the disease or added later to smooth out the Parkinson's disease medication response.

While their effects are generally modest compared to levodopa, they can reduce wearing off and improve consistency of symptom control. Some also appear to have mild benefits for fatigue and mood. The COMT inhibitors are commonly associated with increasing a side effect called dyskinesia. Dyskinesia is a dance-like movement that can emerge, and this may signal a need to reduce the amount of levodopa per dose.

#### THINGS TO KNOW ABOUT THE USE OF MAO-B INHIBITORS

- These drugs have only very small symptomatic effects and they cannot replace levodopa or dopamine agonists.
- These drugs can be used in monotherapy or in combination with other medications.
- To date there has not been overwhelming evidence that these drugs are neuroprotective.
- The risk of an adverse event from mixing a low-dose MAO-B with an antidepressant is very low because it would take high doses of the MAO-B to activate the MAO-A receptor and thus result in the side effects.

#### THINGS TO KNOW ABOUT THE USE OF COMT INHIBITORS

- These medications may extend the effects of a dose of levodopa and can be used between dosages.
- These medications must be taken with carbidopa.
- Frequently, the dose of levodopa and/or agonists must be reduced to avoid dyskinesia when taken with COMT inhibitors.
- Diarrhea and discolored urine are common side effects.

## COMMONLY APPROVED MEDICATIONS FOR PARKINSON'S DISEASE

The following summaries of commonly approved Parkinson's disease medications and their classes are provided for educational purposes. More details on these medications can be found at www.parkinsons.org.

## CURRENTLY APPROVED FOR TREATMENT OF PARKINSON'S DISEASE

| MEDICATION CLASS | MEDICATIONS |
|---|---|
| Carbidopa/levodopa formulations | • Carbidopa/levodopa (Sinemet)<br>• Carbidopa/levodopa orally disintegrating tablet (Parcopa)<br>• Carbidopa/levodopa controlled release (Sinemet CR)<br>• Carbidopa/levodopa/entacapone (Stalevo)<br>• Carbidopa/levodopa extended-release capsules (Rytary)<br>• IPX203 carbidopa/levodopa extended-release capsule (Crexont)<br>Note: This is a gel formulation of the drug that requires a surgically placed tube. |
| Dopamine agonists | • Apomorphine (Apokyn)<br>• Bromocriptine (Parlodel)<br>• Pramipexole (Mirapex)<br>• Pramipexole dihydrochloride extended-release (Mirapex ER)<br>• Ropinirole (Requip)<br>• Ropinirole extended-release tablets (Requip XLTM)<br>• Rotigotine transdermal system (Neupro) |
| COMT inhibitors | • Entacapone (Comtan)<br>• Tolcapone (Tasmar) |
| MAO-B inhibitors | • Rasagiline (Azilect)<br>• Selegiline or deprenyl (Eldepryl)<br>• Selegiline HCl orally disintegrating tablet (Zelapar)<br>• Safinamide (Xadago) |
| Anticholinergics | • Benztropine mesylate (Cogentin)<br>• Procyclidine (not currently available in the U.S.)<br>• Trihexyphenidyl (Artane) |
| Other | • Amantadine extended-release (Gocovri)<br>• Droxidopa (Northera) |
| Istradefylline (Nourianz) | • Rivastigmine (Nuplazid) |

#### Amantadine and other Parkinson's disease medications

Amantadine can help to reduce dyskinesias, which are involuntary movements that may occur after years of disease progression and from levodopa use. Amantadine may also offer modest benefits for tremor and stiffness.

Anticholinergic medications are occasionally used for tremor, particularly in younger folks; however, their cognitive side effects limit use in many individuals. Most experts avoid anticholinergic medications (i.e., Benadryl, trihexyphenidyl) because of the risk of compromised cognitive abilities and the potential increased risk for later dementia.

**DYSKINESIA**

- Dyskinesia refers to involuntary, often flowing or dance-like movements.
- It is commonly related to disease progression and changes in brain sensitivity to dopamine.
- Movements may include writhing, fidgeting, or swaying.
- Dyskinesia frequently appears when medication levels are at their peak.
- It can be bothersome, however it is usually manageable with medication adjustments.

### Motor Fluctuations and Dyskinesia

As Parkinson's progresses, many folks experience fluctuations in how well medications work. Periods when medication is working well are called "on" times. Periods when symptoms return are referred to as "off" times.

Dyskinesia, the involuntary writhing or fidgeting movements, often reflects peaks in dopamine levels. Dyskinesia is associated with disease progression. These movements can be bothersome; however, they are frequently manageable.

Strategies to address fluctuations include adjusting medication timing, using extended-release formulations, adding adjunct medications or considering device-based therapies.

### Advanced Therapies: When Medications Are Not Enough

When medications no longer provide consistent control, advanced therapies can dramatically improve quality of life. These options are underused and may be misunderstood.

#### Deep Brain Stimulation and focused ultrasound therapy

Deep brain stimulation, or DBS, involves implanting thin electrodes into specific brain regions, and these are connected to a pacemaker-like device. Electrical stimulation helps normalize abnormal brain circuits.

DBS can reduce motor fluctuations, dyskinesia, tremor and in some but not all cases reduce medication burden. It does not cure Parkinson's; however, it can restore years of function

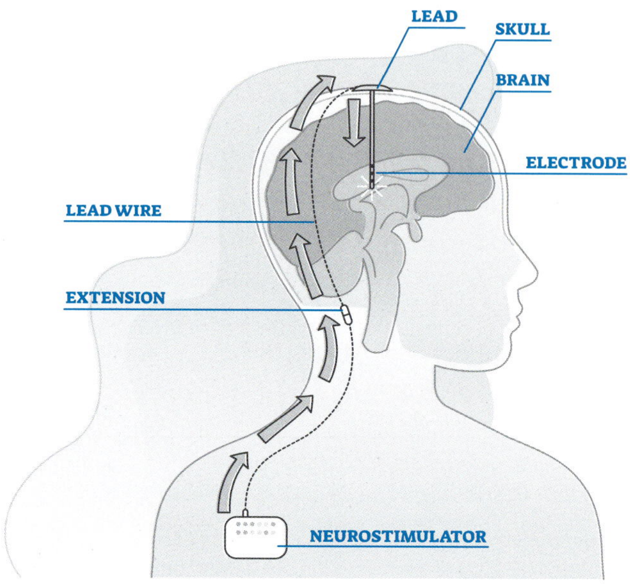


for the right candidate. Timing matters when considering DBS therapy for Parkinson's disease. DBS works best when considered proactively rather than as a last resort. Careful evaluation by an experienced multidisciplinary DBS team is essential.

There is also a second noninvasive procedure called focused ultrasound therapy. This is a therapy that uses sound waves to create lesions in the brain and it can be effective for select persons with Parkinson's disease. The therapy is less precise than DBS, but it does not require an incision or invasive brain surgery.

### Infusion therapies

Continuous infusion of dopaminergic medications through intestinal gel or under the skin may provide a steadier symptom control for select folks with severe fluctuations. These therapies bypass the stomach and thus reduce the variability related to digestion and could reduce food-related interactions. Infusions require commitment and support; however, for some folks they are life-changing.

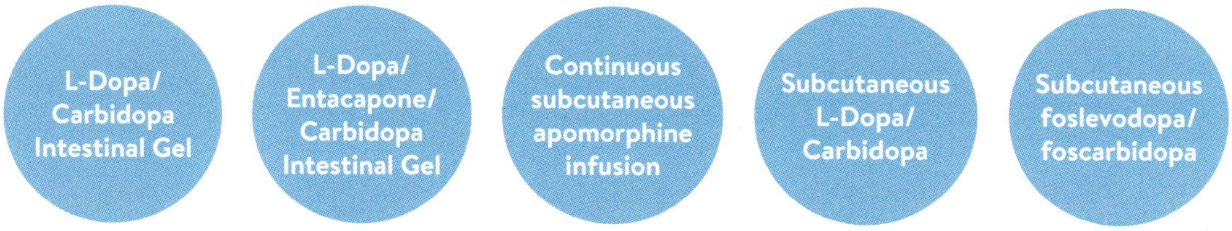

## Rehabilitation: Treating Parkinson's With More than Pills, Infusions and Surgery

Medications alone are not considered enough for the treatment of Parkinson's disease. Most experts and most clinical practice guidelines agree that Parkinson's care must include rehabilitation and movement-based therapies.

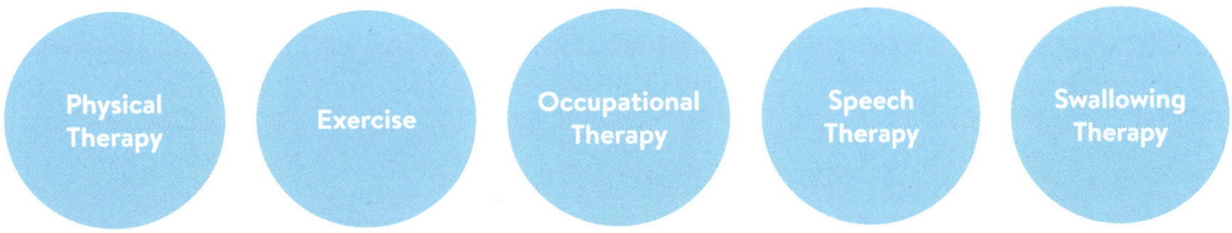


### Physical therapy and exercise

Exercise is medicine for Parkinson's. It improves mobility, balance, strength, mood, sleep and possibly brain health. Structured physical therapy can address gait, posture, freezing and fall risk. Regular aerobic exercise, resistance training, balance work and flexibility exercises should be part of every Parkinson's management plan.

#### WHAT IS THE BEST TYPE OF EXERCISE?

As discussed in this chapter, there are numerous ways to engage in exercise, from indoor to outdoor options, gym programs or group classes, cardiovascular or strengthening, and others. More research is needed to determine which of these is most effective, but the good news is that each has been proven beneficial for people with Parkinson's disease.

Any activity that you engage in daily can help you be successful and slow decline. All exercise is good exercise and the key is consistency. You need to be more active than sedentary and the more intensely you work within reason, the better the results.

Finally, you are more apt to adhere to your exercise routines when you participate in exercise that you enjoy.

### Occupational therapy

Occupational therapists help folks adapt daily activities, conserve energy, improve safety and maintain independence. Small adjustments in how tasks are performed can yield big gains.

### Speech and swallowing therapy

Speech therapy addresses voice volume, clarity and swallowing safety. Programs focused on intensive voice treatment can significantly improve communication and reduce isolation. Swallowing should be regularly checked because the leading cause of death in Parkinson's is aspiration pneumonia. Aspiration pneumonia results from disordered swallowing, which may trigger coughing when eating, leading to infection. There are rehabilitation strategies that can be employed to proactively reduce the risk of aspiration pneumonia.

## Non-Motor Symptoms: The Hidden Burden

Non-motor symptoms often drive disability and distress in Parkinson's disease. These symptoms deserve the same attention as movement problems and they are unfortunately overlooked by many health-care providers.

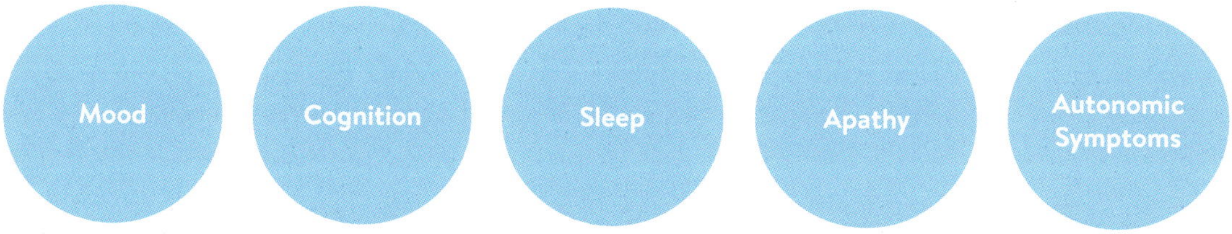


### Mood and anxiety

Depression and anxiety are common and biologically linked to Parkinson's. They are treatable. Counseling, medications, exercise and social connection all play important treatment roles.

### Sleep

Sleep disturbances include insomnia, vivid dreams, REM sleep behavior disorder (acting out dreams) and excessive daytime sleepiness. Addressing sleep improves many other symptoms and improves the ability to live with Parkinson's disease.

### Cognition and thinking

Cognitive changes can be widely variable. Early recognition, cognitive strategies and a review of medications can help preserve function and independence.

## THE CARE TEAM AND THE PARKINSON'S UNIVERSE

Parkinson's is best managed by a team. Neurology specialists, primary care providers, therapists, dietitians, mental health professionals and caregivers all play critical roles.

The person living with Parkinson's remains at the center. Care partners deserve support and education. Community resources, advocacy organizations and peer support all have the potential to strengthen outcomes.

## THE PARKINSON'S UNIVERSE

**ASTEROIDS**
- access
- cost of care
- transportation
- parking
- payers

**MISSION CONTROL**
- coordination of care

**SATELLITES**
- wearables
- telemedicine
- applied A.I.

**STARS**
- support groups
- advocacy groups

**PLUTO**
- stigma

**MERCURY**
- caregiver

**FAMILY, SOCIAL NETWORK, OTHERS WITH PARKINSON'S**

**NEUROLOGIST OR MOVEMENT NEUROLOGIST**

**OTHER MULTIDISCIPLINARY GENERALISTS AND SPECIALISTS**

**ALL PATIENTS**
- caregiver
- specialized practitioner
- general practitioner
- community nurse
- specialized nurse

**MOST PATIENTS**
- psychiatrist
- neuropsychologist
- occupational therapist
- physical therapist
- social worker
- dietitian
- speech therapist

**SOME PATIENTS**
- neurogeneticist
- neuro-ophthalmologist
- rehabilitation therapist
- pulmonologist
- nursing home physician
- occupational physician
- gastroenterologist
- pain specialist
- neurosurgeon
- palliative care team
- pharmacist
- urologist
- sleep specialist
- vascular specialist
- sex therapist
- dentist

### FOOD AND MEDICATION INTERACTIONS

- Protein can compete with levodopa for absorption in the gut and brain.
- This does not mean avoiding protein, it means timing it thoughtfully.
- Taking levodopa on an empty stomach may improve effectiveness for some people.

EXAMPLES

- High-protein meals (e.g., steak, eggs) may reduce medication benefit if taken at the same time.
- Fiber improves gut health and may support medication consistency.
- Hydration supports blood pressure and medication absorption.

**Key principle:** Balance, timing and moderation.

**Autonomic symptoms**

Blood pressure changes, constipation, urinary symptoms and sweating issues are common in Parkinson's disease. These symptoms respond to targeted treatments and lifestyle strategies. Many folks with Parkinson's will experience fainting and passing out and this is frequently mistaken as a heart-related issue when it is really a manifestation of Parkinson's disease.

**Nutrition and medication interactions**

Food influences Parkinson's management in several ways. Protein can compete with levodopa absorption. Hydration affects blood pressure and constipation. Fiber supports gut health. Weight changes influence medication dosing.

The goal of a nutrition program is not restriction. The goal is timing, balance and nourishment. Nutrition should support energy, enjoyment and long-term health while working alongside medications, rather than against them.

## Looking Ahead

Current management strategies for Parkinson's are more powerful than ever before. When used together, they promote living active, meaningful lives sometimes for decades after diagnosis.

This chapter is not about perfection. It is about progress. Parkinson's management should be a proactive living plan, adjusted over time, guided by science and grounded in what matters most to the individual.

The next chapters will build on this foundation, focusing on how nutrition and daily choices can further support health, function and quality of life. Parkinson's may be part of your life; however, it does not have to define your limits.

## References

Cao F, Vogel AP, Gharahkhani P, et al. Speech and language biomarkers for Parkinson's disease prediction, early diagnosis and progression. *NPJ Parkinsons Dis.* 2025 Mar 24;11(1):57. doi: 10.1038/s41531-025-00913-4. PMID: 40128529; PMCID: PMC11933288.

Chaudhary SA, Chaudhary S, Rawat S. Understanding Parkinson's disease: current trends and its multifaceted complications. *Front Aging Neurosci.* 2025 Sep 18;17:1617106. doi: 10.3389/fnagi.2025.1617106. PMID: 41049533; PMCID: PMC12488584.

Langeskov-Christensen M, Franzén E, Grøndahl Hvid L, et al. Exercise as medicine in Parkinson's disease. *J Neurol Neurosurg Psychiatry.* 2024 Oct 16;95(11):1077-1088. doi: 10.1136/jnnp-2023-332974. PMID: 38418216.

Mancini M, Afshari M, Almeida Q, et al. Digital gait biomarkers in Parkinson's disease: susceptibility/risk, progression, response to exercise, and prognosis. *NPJ Parkinsons Dis.* 2025 Mar 21;11(1):51. doi: 10.1038/s41531-025-00897-1. PMID: 40118834; PMCID: PMC11928532.

Müller T. Update on the Present and Future Pharmacologic Treatment of Parkinson's Disease. *Neurol Ther.* 2025 Oct;14(5):1769-1781. doi: 10.1007/s40120-025-00800-3. Epub 2025 Jul 18. PMID: 40679671; PMCID: PMC12450148.

Okun MS, Bloem BR, Dorsey ER. The Parkinson's Universe: A person-centered care model for Parkinson's disease. *J Parkinsons Dis.* 2026 Feb;16(1):192-195. doi: 10.1177/1877718X251399958. Epub 2025 Dec 3. PMID: 41334725.

Okun MS, Malaty IA, Deeb W. *Living with Parkinson's Disease: A Complete Guide for Patients and Caregivers.* Toronto: Robert Rose, 2020.

Peña-Zelayeta L, Delgado-Minjares KM, Villegas-Rojas MM, et al. Redefining Non-Motor Symptoms in Parkinson's Disease. *J Pers Med.* 2025 Apr 26;15(5):172. doi: 10.3390/jpm15050172. PMID: 40423044; PMCID: PMC12112995.

# PART II

# NUTRITION QUALITY OF LIFE IN PARKINSON'S DISEASE

# CHAPTER 3

# NUTRITION AND PARKINSON'S DISEASE

*Understanding the importance of nutrition for overall health will set the stage for Parkinson's disease risk.*

## What Is Nutrition and Why Is It Important?

Nutrition is more than just the food we put on our plates. Nutrition provides a foundation for our bodies to function, grow and repair. The term "nutrition" refers to the combination of protein, carbohydrates, fats, vitamins, minerals and fluids that our bodies need to survive and to thrive. Nutrients provide fuel to the body to carry out basic processes, like pumping blood into vital organs, breathing and moving. Nutrition can also influence mental and emotional well-being by helping to regulate the production of chemical messengers and hormones. The foods we choose can impact sleep, stress and exercise endurance. Nutrition is more than a foundation for general health. Nutrition guides how our bodies will age over time and how susceptible we may be to chronic disease(s).

As people age, their nutritional needs will shift. For example, the factors associated with aging, such as changes in appetite, taste and smell, can all influence the amount of nutrients consumed. Physiological changes, such as altered digestion and shifts in muscle mass, may also influence the amount of nutrients required for health. These factors collectively can make it harder to maintain proper nutrition, even with a balanced diet. Because Parkinson's disease commonly develops in mid-to-late adulthood, the age-related nutrition changes along with the challenges of Parkinson's disease make nutrition an essential component of overall well-being.

While individual nutrients are important, long-term dietary patterns will have a much greater impact on health. A lifestyle that emphasizes whole foods, a balance in ingredients, and moderation will support heart, brain and gut health beyond the use of any single nutrient or supplement. Understanding the importance of nutrition for overall health will set the stage for Parkinson's disease risk and can also impact onset as well as management strategies.

## Science of Parkinson's Disease

A protein called alpha-synuclein (α-syn) is an important component of the Parkinson's disease process. This protein is located at synapses, places where brain cells, or neurons, communicate. α-syn is primarily located in the brain but can be found in smaller amounts in other areas of the body, such as the heart, gut and muscles. This protein aids in communication between cells and α-syn is important in the release of chemicals, like dopamine. When α-syn is at full speed, it supports normal brain signaling.

When α-syn becomes misfolded or has an altered structure, it cannot completely carry out its job. In this scenario, misfolded proteins will begin to clump together, forming debris. This process is thought to impair dopamine release, but it also can lead to damage of the mitochondria, or the energy producers in the brain cells. Mitochondrial dysfunction increases the production of free radicals. Free radicals are tiny, unstable molecules that can damage healthy cells. Free radicals contribute to an imbalance that results in a process called oxidative stress, which is known to further damage brain cells. Neurons affected by this process can become dysfunctional or stop functioning altogether. Neurons in the brain areas that coordinate movement are particularly vulnerable, making this process important to note in the setting of Parkinson's disease.

### UNDERSTANDING OXIDATIVE STRESS

Free radicals are molecules produced naturally by cells. Free radicals are similar to the exhaust produced by a car's engine. A small amount of exhaust is normal; however, if the engine isn't optimally functioning, it will produce an excessive amount of fumes. Excess exhaust is bad for the car and the environment. Similarly, excess free radicals are bad for the brain. Antioxidant foods and drugs act like an emission control system. They can be used to clean up or to reduce the number of free radicals, limiting the amount of exhaust and hopefully heading off damage to the brain cells. When free radical production overwhelms the body's defenses, oxidative stress begins, and this places an added strain on the brain cells affected by Parkinson's disease.

The exact reason why α-syn misfolds remains unknown; however, there are many potential reasons. There may be both genetic and environmental risk factors making it more likely for someone to later develop Parkinson's disease. Additionally, the gut microbiome may be important for risk and progression of Parkinson's disease.

## Gut-Brain Axis

The gut-brain axis refers to the communication pathways between the brain and the gut and in particular the microbiome or organisms that live in your gut. This relationship can influence brain function and overall health. Some experts believe that the gut-brain axis may affect the development and progression of Parkinson's disease, though research on this relationship remains incomplete.

### WHAT IS THE GUT MICROBIOME?

The gut microbiome refers to the diverse environment in the gastrointestinal (GI) tract, also known as the gut. The microbiome is made up of trillions of bacteria, viruses and fungi that can all interact and impact a person's health. Not only are there trillions of microorganisms, but there are also thousands of different *types* of bacteria. These microbes play important roles in:

- Breaking down food
- Promoting regular bowel movements
- Fermenting non-digestible food components
- Maintaining the integrity of the lining of the gastrointestinal tract
- Producing important vitamins and minerals
- Protecting against infection and inflammation

The number and types of bacteria in the gut are influenced by many factors, including diet, age, genetics, physical activity, medication use, environment, stress and sleep.

A balance of good bacteria in the gut produces substances referred to as short-chain fatty acids (SCFAs). These SCFAs help to prevent microbes from leaving the gut by maintaining the integrity of the intestinal lining. SCFAs also help to maintain the strength of the blood-brain barrier (BBB), preventing infectious microbes from crossing into the brain.

### WHAT IS THE BLOOD-BRAIN BARRIER?

The blood-brain barrier (BBB) is a force field surrounding the brain. The BBB acts as a gatekeeper, regulating which substances can enter and exit the brain. The BBB plays an important role in protecting the brain from unwanted infectious diseases and inflammation.

An imbalance in the gut microbiome, termed dysbiosis, has been commonly encountered in persons with Parkinson's disease. This has been referred to as an overgrowth of bad bacteria. These bad bacteria trigger the immune system, leading to inflammation in the entire GI tract. Inflammation is the immune system's response to an injury or infection. Short-term inflammation can be important in healing; however, long-term inflammation can lead to harmful health-related consequences. When long-term inflammation weakens the intestinal lining, it allows microbes to leak out of the GI tract and to travel to other areas of the body.

### PROPOSED ROLE OF THE GUT-BRAIN AXIS IN PARKINSON'S DISEASE

1. An imbalance of gut bacteria triggers an immune response (inflammation) in the gut.
2. Inflammation in the gut weakens the intestinal lining, allowing microbes and inflammatory molecules to leave the gut.
3. This immune response spreads to other areas of the body, causing systemic inflammation.
4. The immune system may respond to areas of the brain (neuroinflammation), possibly triggering misfolding of $\alpha$-syn proteins.

This is referred to as an inflammatory response. An inflammatory response is a chain reaction, triggering inflammation potentially across multiple body systems. When the immune system mounts a response in the brain, it is called neuroinflammation. Neuroinflammation has in some recent research been linked to the misfolding of α-syn proteins, which are known to be highly associated with a diagnosis of Parkinson's disease.

This pathway is only one possible explanation for the onset and progression of Parkinson's disease. Do changes in your gut lead to a diagnosis of Parkinson's disease, or are the changes a result of Parkinson's disease? Or could it be that both are true? Experts believe that gut dysbiosis interacts with genetic, environmental and neurological factors to influence Parkinson's disease. The exact relationships remain to be elucidated.

There is growing evidence supporting gut involvement in Parkinson's disease. GI dysfunction is known to affect over 80% of people living with Parkinson's disease. GI challenges commonly occur long before the appearance of motor symptoms. Symptoms, such as constipation, reduced gut motility and/or swallowing challenges may possibly reflect changes in the gut-brain axis. Additionally, α-syn has been found in the GI tract, including the salivary glands, esophagus, intestines and stomach, suggesting the intriguing possibility that gut involvement may contribute to both motor and non-motor Parkinson's disease symptoms.

## HOW DO YOU KNOW IF YOU HAVE A HEALTHY GUT MICROBIOME?

Microbiome sequencing using a sample of your stool can be used to understand the types and amounts of microbes present in your gut. This test is mostly used in research settings, but it is beginning to appear more commonly during primary care and preventive care visits. Today, your health-care providers rely heavily on signs and symptoms to gauge your gut health. You likely have a healthy gut microbiome if you:

- Have regular bowel movements
- Experience minimal digestive symptoms, such as gas, bloating and abdominal pain
- Can tolerate a range of food groups without adverse symptoms
- Have stable mood and energy levels
- Have a strong immune system

### HOW DO YOU SUPPORT A HEALTHY GUT MICROBIOME?

Factors that foster gut health include a high-fiber diet, regular physical activity, adequate sleep and proactive management of stress. The long-term use of certain medications, low-fiber diets, chronic stress and infections can all disrupt your gut. You can read more about specific diet patterns that support gut health in Chapter 7.

There are likely many factors leading to the development and progression of Parkinson's disease and we should not assume that the gut-brain access is the only factor influencing disease. However, the importance of gut health in Parkinson's disease cannot and should not be overlooked. It is, however, a reasonable conclusion that possessing a balanced gut microbiome will support the integrity of the lining of the GI tract as well as contribute to a stronger BBB. If a balanced gut translates to a strong barrier against neuroinflammation, then a balanced gut microbiome may be important in the holistic treatment of Parkinson's disease.

## Role of Nutrition in Parkinson's Disease Management

In addition to the impact nutrition has on your gut-brain axis, nutrition also may play a key role in managing both motor and non-motor symptoms of Parkinson's disease.

Common non-motor symptoms of Parkinson's disease include constipation, difficulty swallowing and fatigue. These symptoms can be influenced by food choices and by adequate hydration. Nutrition strategies, such as increasing fiber consumption, modifying diet textures and boosting calorie consumption, can all be useful in managing symptoms and improving quality of life.

Adequate hydration is especially important in Parkinson's disease. Proper fluid intake supports normal bowel function, helps maintain blood pressure and can also influence medication absorption. Even mild dehydration can worsen fatigue, trigger dizziness and worsen cognitive function.

People with Parkinson's disease may experience changes in appetite, energy needs and weight. Tremor, rigidity and dyskinesia can increase energy requirements, while swallowing difficulties or nausea can reduce intake.

Eventually, an imbalance can lead to unintended weight loss or malnutrition. These are conditions that can weaken your muscles and compromise your immune function.

Nutrition supports muscle, bone and overall brain health. Certain diet components, such as calcium and vitamin D, support bone strength and are especially important for reducing the risk of fractures related to falling. Balanced meals that include protein, carbohydrates and healthy fats can help to maintain muscle mass and to provide stable energy throughout the course of a day. Additionally, certain dietary patterns rich in fruits, vegetables, whole grains and healthy fats have been associated with better cognitive (thinking) and cardiovascular outcomes.

Nutrition intersects with medication management. Some medications, like levodopa (dopamine replacement therapy), can interact with specific foods, making the timing and composition of meals important treatment considerations if you have Parkinson's disease. Understanding these interactions can in some cases facilitate more optimal control of symptoms.

Nutrition remains at the foundation of your overall health and is especially important in the setting of Parkinson's disease. While no single diet can prevent or cure Parkinson's disease, thoughtful choices in food and adequate hydration have a high potential to improve well-being and enhance quality of life for those living with Parkinson's disease.

### NUTRITION NEEDS

- **Protein:** Supports muscle mass and strength
- **Carbohydrates:** Provide steady energy
- **Healthy fats:** Support brain health (olive oil, nuts, fish)
- **Fiber:** Supports gut health and prevents constipation
- **Calcium + Vitamin D:** Protect bone health
- **Fluids:** Support digestion, blood pressure, and medication response
- **Antioxidants:** Help combat oxidative stress (fruits and vegetables)
- **B vitamins:** Support nerve and brain function (not too much $B_6$)

## Reference

Klann EM, Dissanayake U, Gurrala A, et al. The Gut-Brain Axis and Its Relation to Parkinson's Disease: A Review. *Front Aging Neurosci.* 2022 Jan 7;13:782082. doi: 10.3389/fnagi.2021.782082. PMID: 35069178; PMCID: PMC8776990.

CHAPTER 4

# NON-MOTOR SYMPTOM MANAGEMENT

*Sensory dysfunction impacts not only the amount of food you eat, but also the types of nutrients you consume.*

Non-motor symptoms affect everyone with Parkinson's disease and commonly contribute to quality of life more than the more common classical motor symptoms of the disease. Common non-motor symptoms include gastrointestinal challenges, difficulty swallowing, mood changes, alterations in taste and smell, and changes in blood pressure. Because many of these symptoms directly influence appetite and digestion, they can have a profound impact on both nutritional status and overall well-being. Nutrition strategies have been shown to be important for managing non-motor Parkinson's symptoms.

## Sensory Dysfunction

Changes in smell and taste may be among the first noticeable signs of Parkinson's disease. For some people, a reduced sense of smell can emerge even years before a diagnosis. Because smell and taste are closely connected, if this sense diminishes, it can impact the taste of food. Both taste and smell play important roles in the regulation of appetite. It is well known that when foods appear less flavorful, meals are less enjoyable. Decreased satisfaction with meals is known to be an important driver for a diminished appetite. This can translate to lower overall food intake and unintentional weight loss.

Sensory dysfunction impacts not only the amount of food you eat, but also the types of nutrients you consume. A diminished sense of taste and smell is a frequent reason for people over-seasoning food with salt or for choosing foods with distinct flavors, such as overly sweet foods that are high in sugar. Diminished taste also decreases interest in trying new foods or recipes. Collectively, when one has diminished taste, the diet contains less variety and frequently a paucity of essential nutrients.

Sensory changes are in general not reversible, but there are several nutrition-based strategies that can help to enhance flavor profiles and meal satisfaction:

**1. Enhance the Flavor**
Instead of using salt and sugar to season foods, try using herbs and spices to provide extra flavor without the added negative health consequences. Herbs and spices to consider include basil, thyme, cumin, paprika, ground peppers and blends of curry. Adding acidity by using lemon juice, lime juice or vinegar might provide a flavor pop. Choosing umami flavors, such as those found in mushrooms, some cheeses, miso and soy sauce, can add deeper taste to a bland dish.

**2. Focus on Aroma**
Warm foods tend to emit more aroma than cold foods. Keep this in mind when serving meals, and try to exercise your sense of smell prior to each bite.

**3. Prioritize Other Senses**
When one sense is reduced, lean into your other senses. A focus on texture and visual appeal can transform meals into a more enjoyable experience. Including a variety of textures, such as crispy, creamy and crunchy foods, can enhance the meal. Aiming for a colorful plate has been observed to be helpful. A bland chicken breast, mashed potatoes and white rice appear much less appealing than a glazed barbeque chicken with a bright orange baked sweet potato and steamed green beans.

**4. Experiment with New Foods**
Finding new recipes that utilize bold flavors, such as those with global spice blends, citrus dressings, seasonal produce and fresh herbs, can add to your mealtime experience.

If sensory dysfunction triggers unintentional weight loss, it is critical to address a lack of appetite. When meals become unappealing, focusing on smaller portions eaten more frequently can be helpful. Adding snacks between meals and focusing on nutrient-dense options, such as nuts and nut butters, avocados and olive oil, can make a measurable difference in the experience of a meal. Read more on how to prevent unintentional weight loss later in this chapter.

### MANAGING SENSORY CHANGES

**SIGHT**
- Add color to your meal with vibrant fruits and vegetables or a simple garnish.

**SOUND**
- Mix up crunchy, chewy, hard, and soft foods.

**TASTE**
- Mix up salty, sweet, sour, bitter, and umami. Take time to savor every bite.

**SMELL**
- You may be able to smell warm foods better as they are more aromatic.
- If you have an altered smell that decreases your appetite, lean toward cold foods that are less aromatic.

**TOUCH**
- Use different food textures like crumbly, crunchy, chewy, soft, hard, liquid, and solid.

Other considerations for sensory dysfunction include zinc intake and employing household safety measures:

- For some people, a diminished sense of taste can result from not consuming enough zinc. Women should aim to consume at least 8mg/day of zinc from food sources, and men should aim for at least 11mg/day of zinc from food sources. Food sources of zinc include meat, fish, poultry, whole grains, beans, nuts, and nut butters.
- Zinc supplements in the form of pills can lead to adverse neurological symptoms if overdosed. Most experts recommend not exceeding a total of 40 mg of zinc per day.
- Persistent sensory changes might also lead to safety concerns. If diminished smell affects one's ability to detect gas, odors, smoke, or spoiled foods, household safety measures may need to be implemented.

While there is currently no treatment to fully restore sensory function in Parkinson's disease, several nutrition-based strategies can help to enhance meal satisfaction and improve health. We recommend speaking to your health-care team if sensory dysfunction impacts your quality of life and/or safety.

## Mood and Cognitive Changes

Mood and cognitive changes are common manifestations of Parkinson's disease. Mood and cognitive changes can impact motivation and desire for meal preparation. Some examples of these challenges include depression, anxiety, apathy and mild cognitive impairment or forgetfulness.

Depression and anxiety affect nearly half of people living with Parkinson's disease. These symptoms can manifest as a decreased appetite, a lack of motivation to prepare meals, emotional eating and/or inconsistent patterns of eating. Anxiety may be accompanied by physical symptoms, such as nausea or chest tightness. Depression and anxiety can lead to eating less or eating less frequently. Additionally, people with Parkinson's may choose convenient, less nutritious foods that are easier to prepare, especially when they lack motivation to cook. This scenario can lead to unintentional nutritional deficiencies and weight loss. Emotional eating may have the opposite effect, leading to overeating foods that are high in sugar or sodium. A lack of specific nutrients,

### SNACKS TO SUPPORT STABLE MOOD

- Trail mix
- Granola bar
- Nuts and cheese
- Popcorn
- Peanut butter with fruit
- Rolled oats energy balls
- Tuna or sardines and whole wheat crackers
- Greek yogurt and fruit
- Hummus with pretzels

like fiber, commonly exacerbates non-motor symptoms such as constipation.

Since depression and anxiety are known to impact one's overall nutritional status, it is important to adopt strategies to support a balanced diet. The use of a routine along with a focus on regular, balanced meals can help stabilize blood sugar, energy levels and mood. Including a source of protein, carbohydrates and fat at each meal can provide balance. If lack of motivation to prepare meals is an obstacle, moving to more "convenient food items" with reasonable nutrition content is a powerful strategy. No-cook or quick recipes can help in cases where Parkinson's is accompanied by severe fatigue. When food preparation is challenging, involving family members and friends to assist with tasks such as meal planning, grocery shopping or cooking can be transformative. Finally, pairing cooking and eating with other fun activities, such as listening to music, talking to friends or being outdoors, can make meal preparation and mealtimes more enjoyable.

### NUTRITION STRATEGIES WHEN PARKINSON'S IS ACCOMPANIED BY DEPRESSION AND ANXIETY

1. Establish a meal routine. Aim to eat a balanced meal every 3 to 4 hours. Include a source of protein, carbohydrates and fat at each meal.
2. Use nutrient-rich "convenient foods" when lack of motivation becomes an obstacle. Examples include microwavable whole grains, pre-chopped vegetables, rotisserie chicken, canned fish or easy-to-prepare meal kits.
3. Emphasize low-effort meals when fatigue is burdensome. Try no-cook or 10-minute recipes. Planning ahead by bulk cooking can be helpful for providing easy meals later in the week.
4. Involve your support system to help with various tasks, such as meal planning, grocery shopping, preparing ingredients and cooking.
5. Pair cooking and mealtimes with meaningful activities. Listening to music, enjoying the outdoors and spending time with friends and family can add positivity to your routine.

Cognitive changes can manifest as challenges with planning, organization, multitasking and remembering. These symptoms affect activities of daily living and might impair one's ability to manage a grocery list, plan meals, follow recipes or detect spoiled foods. Without support, meal patterns can become irregular, and one's nutrition status may decline. Common nutrition-related consequences include dehydration from forgetting to drink enough fluids or nutrient deficiencies from under-eating. Finally, addressing safety concerns when handling hot cookware or sharp kitchen tools should always be a priority in the setting of Parkinson's disease.

Nutrition strategies to combat cognitive decline focus on social support, structure and visual cues. Involving loved ones or care partners can be critical elements in staying on track with nutrition and hydration. Care partners can also be called on to assist with grocery shopping or with meal preparation. Establishing predictable routines, such as scheduled meals and snacks, can help to maintain regular caloric intake. Visual cues, such as a posted meal calendar or a list of snack options, can provide not-so-subtle reminders that supporting adequate nutrition is a priority in the treatment of Parkinson's disease. Adding a water bottle in frequently used areas of the home is a helpful strategy to encourage continuous hydration throughout the day.

Mood and cognitive changes often develop gradually and can be overlooked. Recognizing symptoms early and taking a proactive approach ensures individuals receive support. While nutrition alone cannot prevent or reverse mood and cognitive changes in Parkinson's disease, thoughtful dietary strategies paired with optimization of medication, mental health support and regular cognitive stimulation can all promote well-being.

### HOW CARE PARTNERS CAN SUPPORT LOVED ONES WITH COGNITIVE CHANGES

- Help with meal planning by gathering recipes
- Help with grocery shopping by making a grocery list and/or assisting during grocery shopping
- Help with ingredient preparation, assembly, and/or cooking
- Stock convenient snacks in an accessible location
- Provide gentle reminders to eat and/or drink
- Use visual cues, such as a calendar with a meal plan and/or sticky notes with reminders
- Assess safety around heating elements and sharp kitchen items
- Exercise patience with yourself and your loved one

## Gastrointestinal Problems

**Constipation** is a common non-motor symptom in Parkinson's disease. Constipation affects an estimated 50% to 80%, and for many, constipation symptoms can begin up to 20 years before Parkinson's-related motor symptoms are recognized. Chronic constipation has been linked to an increased risk for later developing Parkinson's disease. The Honolulu Heart and Aging Study revealed that males aged 51 to 75 years with less than one bowel movement per day were 2.7 times more likely to later develop Parkinson's disease when compared to those that had at least one bowel movement per day. Constipation in Parkinson's disease is thought to be driven by slowed movement of the intestine. This slowed motility paired with Parkinson's-related changes such as reduced physical activity, alterations in gut bacteria, side effects from medications, and inadequate fluid or fiber intake makes constipation a formidable challenge.

## WHAT IS CONSTIPATION?

Constipation can be diagnosed using many different criteria, which makes estimating the number of people who experience constipation hard to pinpoint. The Rome IV criteria for functional constipation is commonly used to diagnose constipation in the setting of Parkinson's disease. According to these criteria, constipation is present when:

1. An individual experiences at least 2 of the following symptoms:
   - Straining
   - Hard or lumpy stools
   - Sensation of incomplete evacuation or anorectal blockage
   - Need for manual assistance during defecation
   - Fewer than 3 spontaneous bowel movements per week
2. These symptoms are experienced for at least 25% of defecations for the past 3 months, with symptom onset at least 6 months prior to diagnosis.

Constipation can impact one's overall nutritional status, and it is commonly accompanied by bloating, nausea and early fullness. These symptoms can become compounded because it becomes progressively more challenging to eat enough throughout the course of a day. Constipation can lead to a lower intake of crucial nutrients. Constipation can also impact the way medications are absorbed. If gastric emptying is delayed or inconsistent, levodopa might not be absorbed in a timely manner, leading to motor symptom fluctuations. Managing constipation is not only important for comfort and for maintaining good nutrition, it is also important for supporting predictable motor symptom control in the setting of Parkinson's disease.

Dietary fiber and fluid intake are important for promoting regular bowel movements. Dietary fiber is a carbohydrate that the body cannot digest or absorb. It travels through the digestive tract, adds bulk to stool and helps stool to retain fluid which encourages it to more efficiently transit the intestines. Most adults should aim to consume 25 to 38 grams of daily fiber. Data strongly suggests that more than 90% of women and 97% of men do not meet recommended intakes for dietary fiber. Further, more than 85% of adults under-consume fruits, vegetables and whole grains, which are the primary sources of fiber in the diet.

### HIGH-FIBER FOODS

- Apples
- Avocado
- Beans
- Berries
- Kiwifruit
- Leafy greens
- Lentils
- Oatmeal
- Pears
- Peas
- Popcorn
- Quinoa
- Seeds (flax, chia)
- Shredded wheat cereal
- Wheat bran

When incorporating more fiber into the diet, it is important to do so gradually. Adding too much fiber, too fast, may lead to abdominal discomfort, gas and bloating. Drinking plenty of water is an important adjunct to increasing fiber intake. Most adults should aim for at least 8 cups (2 L) of water per day.

### TIPS FOR INCREASING FIBER INTAKE AND PROMOTING REGULAR BOWEL MOVEMENTS:

1. When baking, use whole wheat flour instead of white flour.
2. Start your day with a high-fiber cereal, such as shredded wheats or oatmeal. Add a few tablespoons (30 mL) of wheat bran to the mix for a boost of fiber.
3. Add beans to soups and stews. Not only do they provide fiber, but they also provide a plant-based source of protein.
4. Opt for high-fiber snacks, such as fruits and vegetables. Aim for at least 5 servings of fruits and vegetables per day.
5. Eat consistently and avoid skipping meals. This helps keep the GI tract moving throughout the day.
6. Stay physically active to help stimulate GI movement. Work with a physical therapist to understand which movements are safe for you.
7. Drink at least 8 cups (2 L) of water throughout the day, unless your health-care provider advises "less is more."

## A FOCUS ON FRUIT

Fruit is effective for managing constipation symptoms. Many fruits have a combination of soluble and insoluble fiber. Additionally, they have naturally occurring sugars that work together with fiber to draw water into the intestine and to soften the stool. Using fruit can be helpful in managing slow transit constipation because the longer the stool stays in the intestine, the more dehydrated it can become. Dehydrated stool, or dry and lumpy stool, is more difficult to push out and can lead to straining. Some fruits are better than others at managing constipation:

**1. Prunes and Prune Juice**

Some studies show prunes increase stool output and may help balance gut bacteria.

**2. Kiwifruit**

Some studies show two kiwifruits per day could decrease gut transit time and increase the water content of stool, leading to more regular, softer stools for individuals experiencing constipation.

**3. Berries**

Raspberries, blackberries and blueberries are great sources of fiber and polyphenols. These components promote beneficial gut bacteria that could support regular bowel movements.

While constipation in Parkinson's disease is common, severe or persistent symptoms should be evaluated. Fiber supplements and medications, like stool softeners and laxatives, may be appropriate if diet modifications do not improve constipation symptoms. Be sure to talk to your health-care team about whether additional testing is needed.

**Gastroparesis**, or delayed gastric emptying, occurs when the stomach fails to empty foods into the intestine at a rate compatible with normal digestion. The symptoms of gastroparesis may include nausea, vomiting, abdominal pain, bloating and/or feelings of fullness after eating. This condition is diagnosed via what is called a gastric emptying study. During this test, a person eats a small portion of food that is labeled with a special tracer. Imaging is used to track the tracer contained in the food to determine how long it will take for the food to be digested and emptied into the intestines.

Gastroparesis affects an estimated 45% of people living with Parkinson's disease, and its frequency is higher as the disease advances. Gastroparesis is a condition that can lead to unintentional weight loss, malnutrition and poor quality of life. Not only can it cause unwanted symptoms and lead to nutritional concerns, but it can also delay the absorption of antiparkinsonian medications, potentially leading to more on-off times.

The nutrition-based strategies for managing gastroparesis include modifying food textures, changing the contents and sizes of meals, and adjusting meal timing. Imagine a kitchen blender that is always set to the on position. When larger, fibrous foods, like whole apples, are placed in the blender, it will take longer to completely blend the food. In comparison, if pre-blended or less fibrous foods, like applesauce, are placed in the blender, the blender does not have to work as hard and the job is completed more rapidly. The stomach works in a similar way. Softer, less fibrous foods lead to less adverse symptoms as the stomach can empty them faster.

### WHAT IS GASTROPARESIS?

Gastroparesis is when the stomach digests food slowly leading to nausea, vomiting, and early fullness. If untreated, it can lead to unintentional weight loss and even malnutrition. Modifying food textures and meal timing can help the stomach digest food more efficiently.

## TIPS FOR MANAGING GASTROPARESIS

**1. Modify Food Textures**

Choose softer foods that are easier to digest. These foods might include ground meat and poultry, fish, eggs, vegetables cooked well and canned fruits. Avoid tough meats (e.g., steak), raw vegetables and tough fruits. Be cautious with high-fiber foods, such as whole grains, beans and nuts. Be sure to chew foods well before swallowing. Liquid foods, such as commercial nutrition drinks, homemade smoothies or soups, may be better tolerated, especially later in the day.

**2. Limit Fatty Foods**

Foods higher in fat take longer to digest. Limit fried foods, solid fats (e.g., butter, lard, chicken skin, meat gristle) and full-fat dairy products. Instead choose liquid fats for cooking (e.g., oils) and opt for low-fat dairy products (such as 1% and 2% milk, low-fat ice cream and low-fat cheese).

**3. Adjust Meal Sizes and Timing**

Eat smaller, frequent meals to give your stomach less to digest at one time while still meeting your nutrition needs. Instead of eating 3 big meals per day, aim for 5-6 smaller meals and snacks.

| 1-DAY MEAL PLAN ON A REGULAR DIET | 1-DAY MEAL PLAN FOR GASTROPARESIS |
|---|---|
| **BREAKFAST**<br>• Breakfast sandwich (English muffin, 1 fried egg, 1 turkey sausage patty, 1 slice Cheddar cheese, raw spinach, 1 slice tomato)<br>• Apple slices | **BREAKFAST**<br>• Omelet with cooked spinach and diced tomato<br>• Grits<br>• Canned peaches |
| | **SNACK**<br>• Low-fiber oral nutrition supplement |
| **LUNCH**<br>• Tuna sandwich (whole wheat bread, canned tuna, mayonnaise)<br>• Celery and carrots with ranch dressing<br>• Fresh mixed berries | **LUNCH**<br>• ½ tuna sandwich (white bread, canned tuna, small amount of low-fat mayonnaise)<br>• Fruit cup |
| **SNACK**<br>• Almonds<br>• Whole wheat crackers<br>• Cheese cubes | **SNACK**<br>• Small smoothie (low-fat strawberry Greek yogurt, banana, low-fat milk) |
| **DINNER**<br>• Steak<br>• Salad with dressing<br>• Sweet potato with butter | **DINNER**<br>• Ground chicken<br>• Low-sodium canned green beans<br>• ½ sweet potato cooked soft without the skin |

**Nausea and vomiting** can occur due to delayed stomach emptying, medication side effects, dehydration and constipation. Understanding the root cause is the first step in managing these symptoms. If nausea and vomiting go unmanaged, they can lead to inadequate food intake, weight loss and malnutrition.

Nutrition strategies, such as taking medications with food, focusing on specific types of foods and maintaining adequate hydration, may help to reduce nausea and vomiting.

- If taking levodopa on an empty stomach leads to nausea, one could try taking it with a bland carbohydrate such as crackers, toast or applesauce. For those concerned about an interaction between the medication and food, read more on medication-diet interactions in Chapter 5.
- If nausea and vomiting occur due to delayed stomach emptying, try to avoid meals high in fat, which can delay digestion. See this chapter's section on gastroparesis (page 48) for more strategies.

- Focusing on the content of meals can also help prevent nausea. Cold foods tend to be less aromatic and easier to eat when nausea occurs. Small, frequent meals might be easier to eat when feeling sick.
- Ginger can in some cases help to relieve nausea. Fresh ginger can be added to foods or smoothies. Products like ginger tea or ginger candies might also be helpful.
- Staying hydrated can be important for reducing nausea and vomiting. Of course, drinking water is important; however, flavored fluids, such as electrolyte drinks, ice pop or broths, might be easier to handle when feeling nauseous.

If nausea or vomiting affect your ability to consume enough food throughout the day, be sure to talk to your health-care team to understand the underlying cause and discuss treatment options. It is important to address these symptoms early to prevent further nutrition-related concerns.

## Swallowing Difficulty (Dysphagia)

People living with Parkinson's disease may have trouble swallowing at any stage of the disease. The clinical term for swallowing difficulty is "dysphagia." Dysphagia affects more than 80% of people living with Parkinson's disease, and it can increase one's risk for choking, or aspiration. Choking can lead to bacterial growth in the lungs, termed pneumonia. This can lead to sickness and in some cases even death, especially in the elderly population.

Dysphagia increases the risk for malnutrition. Since swallowing might take more effort, dysphagia may also lead to fatigue during eating. People with dysphagia may take longer to eat a meal, resulting in them not being able to finish all their food. When paired with other common Parkinson's symptoms, such as changes in taste and appetite, dysphagia can contribute to poor nutritional status.

### CAN YOU TELL IF YOU HAVE TROUBLE SWALLOWING?

Many people do not realize they have swallowing dysfunction. Ask your doctor if they feel you should have a swallow evaluation. During a swallow evaluation, a speech-language pathologist (SLP) uses imaging to evaluate how well you swallow various consistencies of food. The SLP can make recommendations about which diet textures may be safest to eat and can provide strategies to help you improve your swallowing function.

There are many strategies to make swallowing safer, including working with a doctor to optimize medications, implementing swallowing therapy with an SLP or speaking with a registered dietitian (RD) about making changes to the diet. The first line of treatment for dysphagia from a nutrition perspective is the use of oral nutrition supplements and texture-modified diets.

- Oral nutrition supplements, commonly known as nutrition shakes or protein shakes, are great ways to add calories and protein to a diet. There are many brands and flavors available, all providing different amounts of nutrients. These products can be consumed with meals or as a snack between meals. A registered dietitian can help determine which product might be best for you.
- Texture-modified diets may be used to make foods easier to chew and to swallow. An SLP can help determine which diet is the best fit. Since changes to diet texture may lead to reduced calorie, protein and fiber consumption, an RD can help ensure one is meeting nutrition needs during dietary changes.

## Types of Texture-Modified Diets

A **Regular Easy-to-Chew** diet is recommended if you prefer softer foods or have mouth or jaw pain. This diet is not recommended for swallowing difficulty or for people at a higher risk for choking. Foods not on a regular easy-to-chew diet include those that are hard, dry, tough, crispy, crunchy, sharp, stringy, sticky or gummy.

### EXAMPLES OF REGULAR EASY-TO-CHEW FOODS

- Moistened cereals (e.g., oatmeal)
- Rice, pasta and bread that can be broken into smaller pieces
- Tender red meats, poultry, seafood and deli meats
- Eggs, meat alternatives, beans and lentils
- Milk, yogurt, cottage cheese and pudding
- Soft cooked vegetables
- Canned, cooked and soft fruits (e.g., peaches, kiwi, honeydew and strawberries)

A **Soft and Bite-Size** diet is recommended for someone who has trouble biting off pieces of food but is able to chew the pieces and swallow them in a safe fashion. Food particles should be no larger than 0.6 inches square (1.5 cm square), or about the width of a standard dinner fork. Foods not on a soft and bite-size diet include dry grains, whole nuts and seeds, beans and lentils with hard shells or skins, hard or dry cheeses, raw and fibrous vegetables, dried fruits, and foods where the solid separates from the liquid (e.g., beef stew).

## EXAMPLES OF SOFT AND BITE-SIZE FOODS

- Moistened cereals served without excess liquid (e.g., strained cereal)
- Rice served with thick sauce to prevent the pieces from separating
- Tender red meats and poultry chopped into bite-size pieces
- Yogurt, cottage cheese and soft cheeses
- Soft cooked vegetables served in bite-size pieces
- Canned, cooked and soft fruits, with excess liquid drained off

A **Minced and Moist** diet is recommended if you are unable to bite food, have difficulty chewing food or you get tired when eating. Foods should be minced, soft and moist. Food pieces should be no larger than 0.59 by 0.15 inches (15 by 4 mm) long. Foods not on this diet include dried breads, noodles with sizes that do not meet size requirements, poultry or fish with skin or bones, whole nuts and seeds, raw vegetables, dried fruits and most fresh fruit with peels or seeds.

## EXAMPLES OF MINCED AND MOIST FOODS

- Soft cooked pasta that meets size requirements
- Cooked, moist, soft and tender meats that are minced or mashed
- Yogurt, mashed cottage cheese and pudding
- Cooked tender vegetables
- Canned and cooked fruits drained of excess liquid
- Soft, peeled fresh fruit (e.g., peaches, kiwi)

A **Puréed** diet is recommended if you are unable to bite or chew food or have difficulty swallowing. Foods should be smooth and free of lumps. These foods do not require chewing. Foods not on a puréed diet include foods with lumps, nut butters and jellies, raw or fried vegetables, and non-puréed or stringy fruits.

## EXAMPLES OF PURÉED FOODS

- Puréed hot cereals (e.g., oatmeal)
- Puréed pasta, rice or potatoes without lumps
- Puréed meats, eggs, soft foods and legumes
- Smooth yogurt and whipped cream cheese
- Puréed vegetables
- Smooth tomato sauce and whipped sweet potatoes
- Puréed canned or cooked fruit, drained of excess liquid (e.g., applesauce)

If a person living with Parkinson's disease has significant swallowing difficulty that is preventing them from meeting their nutrition needs by mouth, a feeding tube may be considered. The most common type of long-term feeding tube is called a gastrostomy tube, or g-tube. A g-tube provides a way to deliver nutrition, hydration and/or medications directly into the stomach or intestine. It's typically placed in an outpatient setting, and recovery time is relatively short.

Since swallowing difficulty is a common non-motor symptom and can lead to poor nutrition status, it is important for patients living with Parkinson's disease to notify their health-care team if they notice changes in weight. Early signs of swallowing difficulty can include coughing when eating or drinking or feeling as if foods become stuck when swallowing. Early intervention with texture-modified diets and swallow therapy could make swallowing both easier and safer.

## FREQUENTLY ASKED QUESTIONS ABOUT FEEDING TUBES

**Will a feeding tube prevent me from eating?**

People with feeding tubes are still able to eat by mouth if it is safe to do so. For example, if one can swallow puréed foods safely but they are unable to eat enough puréed foods to maintain their weight, they may use a feeding tube to supplement the nutrition they are not receiving by mouth.

**What goes in the feeding tube?**

A feeding tube can be used for water, medications and nutrition. Using water flushes through the tube can be important for hydration. Some medications can be crushed and administered through the tube, but be sure to check with a doctor or pharmacist before crushing medications. Nutrition can also be delivered through the tube using tube feeding formula. Tube feeding formula has a similar look and consistency of a commercial protein shake and is specially formulated to meet the nutrition needs of an individual. A registered dietitian (RD) will help determine the best formula for each person.

**Is a feeding tube permanent?**

A feeding tube can be removed if it is no longer being used. However, since Parkinson's disease is a progressive disease, it is more likely that the feeding tube will continue to be used as swallowing function declines.

**What are the risks?**

Potential risks include infection, minor pain and discomfort after initial placement, and anesthesia risks.

## Unintentional Weight Loss and Malnutrition

Unintentional weight loss is a frequent and significant concern in Parkinson's disease. Weight loss happens when one does not take in enough nutrition to keep up with the body's energy demands. Not only does the body burn energy when physically active, but even at rest, basic metabolic processes, such as breathing and blood circulation, require a substantial amount of energy. Some studies suggest people living with Parkinson's disease may require more energy than their healthy counterparts. Although not fully understood, this increase in energy requirements may stem from greater physical demands, particularly in the presence of tremors or dyskinesias. Increased energy requirements also may result from changes in the way your body's cells use and produce energy.

Beyond potential increases in energy needs, people living with Parkinson's disease often face multiple challenges that influence how much nutrition they can consume. Motor symptoms such as tremor, rigidity and postural instability can make preparing meals, chewing and feeding oneself more difficult, frequently resulting in reduced caloric intake over time. Non-motor symptoms, including constipation, gastroparesis, dysphagia and mood changes, might further affect appetite, comfort and food choices. For people taking levodopa, meal timing can be complex, and concerns about protein interactions could lead to the avoidance of potentially more nutritious foods.

### WHAT IS AN APPROPRIATE WEIGHT?

Body mass index (BMI) uses your height and weight to estimate your total body composition. Using a BMI chart can help determine if your BMI is in the normal range. However, BMI only tells one part of the story, as it does not consider fat and fat-free mass, including muscle mass. BMI interpretations should be used with caution, especially in older adults and people living with chronic diseases, as these conditions might affect body composition. Optimal BMI ranges increase with your age. Your health-care team can help to determine a healthy weight range based on your medical history, body composition and lifestyle.

## WHY WEIGHT LOSS HAPPENS IN PARKINSON'S DISEASE

| REASON | CONTRIBUTING FACTORS | OUTCOME |
|---|---|---|
| Increased Energy Needs | • Tremor<br>• Dyskinesia<br>• Muscle rigidity<br>• Altered metabolism | • Higher calorie expenditure makes it harder to meet nutrition needs through a normal diet |
| Chewing or Swallowing Problems (Dysphagia) | • Poor oral motor coordination<br>• Muscle rigidity<br>• Slowed swallow reflex | • Avoidance of certain food textures<br>• Longer mealtimes<br>• Increased risk of choking<br>• Inadequate nutrient intake |
| Gastrointestinal Dysfunction | • Constipation<br>• Gastroparesis<br>• Nausea and vomiting<br>• Bloating<br>• Reflux | • Reduced appetite and decreased food intake due to fullness and discomfort |
| Mood Changes | • Depression<br>• Anxiety<br>• Apathy | • Decreased interest in food<br>• Lack of motivation to cook or eat |
| Reduced Appetite and Early Satiety | • Depression and anxiety<br>• Gastroparesis<br>• Nausea<br>• Medication side effects | • Decreased food intake<br>• Unintentional meal skipping |
| Sensory Changes | • Diminished sense of smell<br>• Reduced taste perception | • Less enjoyment of food<br>• Decreased appetite<br>• Reduced overall food intake<br>• Less diet variety |
| Difficulty Eating | • Bradykinesia<br>• Tremor<br>• Hand weakness<br>• Difficulty using utensils<br>• Fatigue | • Difficulty feeding oneself can lead to smaller portions eaten<br>• Early meal termination<br>• Longer mealtimes |
| Medication Timing and Food Interactions | • Nausea from medications<br>• Levodopa–dietary protein interaction | • Disrupted eating patterns<br>• Reduced intake<br>• Food avoidance |
| Cognitive Changes | • Forgetfulness<br>• Difficulty planning meals<br>• Impaired decision-making<br>• Reduced initiative | • Meal skipping<br>• Irregular eating patterns |
| Social Isolation | • Eating alone<br>• Reduced social engagement during mealtimes | • Decreased appetite<br>• Fewer structured meals |

Weight loss is an indicator for malnutrition. Malnutrition results from a lack of adequate calories, protein or other nutrients needed for tissue maintenance and repair. Estimates suggest that up to 24% of people living with Parkinson's disease may already be malnourished, and as many as 60% may be at risk. Malnutrition is also closely linked to sarcopenia, which is a loss of muscle, strength and physical function that is particularly concerning in older adults. Together, these conditions increase the risk of falls, make recovery from illness more difficult and prolonged, and can raise the likelihood of hospitalization. Malnutrition is associated with reduced functional ability, diminished independence and lower overall quality of life.

Fortunately, nutrition interventions can be highly effective in preventing and addressing malnutrition. Strategies may include following a high-calorie, high-protein diet, adjusting meal timing, modifying food textures and incorporating nutrient-dense snacks throughout the day.

## HIGH-CALORIE, HIGH-PROTEIN SNACK IDEAS

- Cottage cheese with pineapple, peaches or grape tomatoes
- Peanut butter toast with banana slices
- Apple slices with peanut butter
- Avocado toast
- Bagel with cream cheese
- Tuna salad with crackers
- Greek yogurt with strawberries and granola
- Milk mixed with protein powder
- Smoothie made with nut butter, milk and fruit

Weight loss leading to malnutrition can occur gradually, so it is important to keep an eye on your body weight trends. If you notice weight loss and cannot identify a reason why, such as increased physical activity, recent illness or intentionally limiting food intake, this is called unintentional weight loss. It is important to mention any changes in weight to your health-care team so that early interventions can be discussed.

## HIGH-CALORIE, HIGH-PROTEIN DIET

A diet high in calories and protein may be recommended to prevent weight loss or to promote gradual weight gain. This diet focuses on foods that are nutrient-dense to meet nutritional needs. In addition to including nutrient-dense foods at every meal, this diet also includes strategies, such as adjustments to food textures and meal timing, to encourage a higher overall intake of food.

### High-Protein Foods

- Meats (beef, pork, venison, buffalo, etc.)
- Poultry (chicken, turkey, etc.)
- Fish (salmon, tuna, sardines, etc.)
- Dairy products (milk, yogurt, cheese, etc.)
- Eggs
- Beans, peas and lentils
- Nuts, nut butters and seeds
- Commercial protein drinks (protein content can vary)

### High-Calorie Foods

- Oils and butters
- Creams, sauces and gravies
- Avocados and olives
- Nuts, nut butters and seeds
- Fatty fish (salmon, tuna, sardines, etc.)
- Commercial protein drinks (look for "plus" options, which are higher in calories)

### Strategies

- Eat smaller, more frequent meals (3 meals and 3 snacks daily)
- Focus on liquid nutrition when appetite is poor (commercial nutrition drinks, homemade smoothies or milkshakes)
- Add oils, butter or gravies to meals
- Drink milk instead of water with meals
- Eat cottage cheese or yogurt with fruit
- Add nut butters to toast, crackers, fruit or smoothies
- Add protein powder to baked goods (like muffins) and smoothies

## Orthostatic Hypotension

Some people living with Parkinson's disease experience changes in blood pressure, termed orthostatic hypotension. Orthostatic hypotension occurs when someone's blood pressure drops significantly upon standing up from a sitting or lying down position. Common symptoms include fainting or lightheadedness, vision changes, cognitive impairment, shortness of breath and/or fatigue. Some patients may not experience symptoms but may still be at an increased risk for injuries and falls.

Some people notice blood pressure changes following a meal. This is because blood pools in the abdominal area during digestion. People that experience fainting, lightheadedness, vision changes or sleepiness after meals may have what is called postprandial hypotension.

For both conditions, there are medication and lifestyle changes that may be helpful. Lifestyle changes might include avoiding certain movements and positions. Nutrition interventions might include focusing on hydration, increasing salt consumption and modifying the content of meals. It is best to work with your health-care team, including your neurologist, physical therapists and dietitians, to comprehensively manage your blood pressure if you experience these symptoms.

### STRATEGIES FOR INCREASING WATER AND SALT CONSUMPTION:

1. Start your day with 2 cups (500 mL) of water. Studies show that drinking 2 cups of water can help increase blood pressure within 30 to 90 minutes.
2. Drink broths and eat soups made with full-sodium broths.
3. Drink sugar-free or low-sugar electrolyte or "sports" drinks. Add electrolyte powders to water.
4. Focus on high-sodium foods, such as canned items or salted nuts and seeds.
5. Set a timer as a reminder to drink fluids throughout the day.
6. Consume salt tablets if needed. These typically have 0.5 to 1 gram of sodium per tablet.

### NUTRITION INTERVENTIONS FOR ORTHOSTATIC HYPOTENSION*

1. Increase water intake to up to 10.5 cups (2.5 L) daily.
2. Increase salt intake to at least 2 to 3 grams daily and up to 6 to 10 grams daily.
3. Drink 2 cups (500 mL) of water upon waking up, before getting out of bed in the morning.

*Use caution if you have heart, kidney or liver failure.

For postprandial hypotension, modification of meals may be necessary. Studies show the size of a meal and the carbohydrate content can affect blood pressure. It is best to aim for 5 to 6 small meals and snacks throughout the day rather than 3 large meals. Reducing alcohol consumption can also help to stabilize blood pressure in some cases. You may also be advised to avoid standing or physical activity directly after a meal.

### NUTRITION INTERVENTIONS FOR POSTPRANDIAL HYPOTENSION

1. Avoid large meals. Instead eat 5 to 6 smaller meals and snacks throughout the day.
2. Aim for less than 65 grams of carbohydrates at meals. Examples of carbohydrate-rich foods include breads, pastas, tortillas, rice, potatoes and corn. Sugary items, like desserts and sugar-sweetened beverages, are also high in carbohydrates.
3. Opt for foods at lower temperatures when possible. Consuming higher-temperature foods may lower blood pressure.
4. Reduce alcohol consumption.

## Osteoporosis

Osteoporosis is a bone disease characterized by low bone density, which increases the likelihood of fractures. Bone loss can progress silently for many years without symptoms, which makes early prevention important especially as people age. Multiple factors, including poor calcium and vitamin D intake, reduced mobility and natural changes in bone metabolism, all contribute to the progression of osteoporosis.

People living with Parkinson's disease have twice the risk for developing osteoporosis, and several factors contribute to this vulnerability. Diet and appetite changes might influence one's ability to consume enough vitamin D and calcium. Low body weight, which is more common for those with Parkinson's disease, is also associated with decreased bone density. Additionally, weight-bearing exercise plays a vital role in building and maintaining strong bones, but symptoms like muscle rigidity, balance changes and freezing episodes may limit a person's ability to stay active. These changes in movement also increase the risk of falls, meaning that weakened bones and increased fall frequency together can significantly increase fracture risk. Men are also at twice the risk of osteoporosis with Parkinson's disease.

### DOUBLE WHAMMY: OSTEOPOROSIS RISK IN POST MENOPAUSAL WOMEN WITH PARKINSON'S DISEASE

Estrogen is a hormone that plays a vital role in maintaining bone health. It helps with calcium absorption and bone remodeling. Estrogen levels can fall dramatically during and after menopause, leading to a higher risk for bone disease. In fact, a 3% to 5% reduction in bone mass can occur each year during the first five years after menopause. Postmenopausal women living with Parkinson's disease are at a higher risk for developing osteoporosis.

Several nutrients and key dietary habits can help to support bone strength and reduce fracture risk. Understanding these nutrition strategies can help people living with Parkinson's disease be proactive in preventing osteoporosis.

- Consuming plenty of **calcium** supports bone health. Calcium is the primary mineral in bone. Adults generally need 1,000 mg per day; however, these needs increase to 1,200 mg per day in women over the age of 50 and men over the age of 70. Dairy is a great source of calcium and includes foods like milk, yogurt and cheese. Other non-dairy foods high in calcium include canned fish with bones, tofu, dark green vegetables and almonds. Many foods are fortified with calcium, meaning additional calcium is added to the food. Examples of foods fortified with calcium include fruit juices, cereals and milk substitutes.
- Consuming plenty of **vitamin D** helps the body absorb calcium and supports muscle function. Low vitamin D levels are common in people living with Parkinson's disease due to limited sun exposure, poor dietary intake and a decline in vitamin D synthesis with age. Adults generally need 15 mcg of vitamin D per day, and this number increases to 20 mcg per day after the age of 70. Vitamin D is found naturally in fatty fish, cod liver oil, beef liver, egg yolks and mushrooms. Fortified foods also provide vitamin D, and these foods include milk and milk alternatives, cheese, ice cream, yogurt, breakfast cereals and orange juice. Supplements are also available for those who are not able to maintain adequate levels of vitamin D with diet and sun exposure.
- Adequate **protein** intake is essential for maintaining muscle mass and supporting bone remodeling. If poor appetite or swallowing difficulty is present, meeting daily protein needs might prove challenging. Incorporating protein at every meal can help maintain strength and reduce the risk of falling. Adults generally need 0.8 grams of protein per *kilogram* of body weight (about 1.8 g/lb). However, this recommendation changes with age and with certain medical conditions. It is best to discuss individual protein needs with a registered dietitian. Protein sources may include meats, poultry, fish, dairy products, eggs, beans, lentils, nuts and meat alternatives.

## VITAMINS: FOOD VS SUPPLEMENTS

- Food is generally the best source of vitamins.
- Whole foods provide nutrients plus fiber and beneficial compounds.
- Supplements may be helpful when deficiencies are present.
- Calcium and vitamin D are especially important for bone health.
- A food-first approach is preferred, with supplements used strategically.

## WATCH YOUR SALT INTAKE

Consuming too much salt (sodium) can cause your body to get rid of too much calcium through urine. It is important to eat plenty of calcium-rich foods while being mindful of your sodium consumption. Most adults should limit their salt intake to less than 2,300mg per day. Foods high in sodium include:

- Ultra-processed foods, such as potato chips and crackers
- Cured and luncheon meats, like salami and ham
- Canned soups and vegetables
- Fast food, including pizza
- Pickled foods
- Condiments, gravies, and dressings
- Boxed meals and casseroles

- Eating plenty of **fruits and vegetables** also supplies essential vitamins and minerals that can support bone health. Nutrients like magnesium, potassium and vitamin A are commonly found in produce and are linked with better bone density. Most adults should aim for at least 2½ cups (625 mL) of vegetables and 2 cups (500 mL) of fruit each day.
- **Limiting high-sodium foods,** like fast food, canned soups, cured meats and other highly-processed items, can help to support bone health along with other nutrition strategies. Too much sodium along with not enough calcium can exacerbate bone loss.

While nutrition and exercise are important for maintaining bone health, they are unlikely to increase bone density alone, especially once osteoporosis has been diagnosed. Health-care providers might recommend medications along with adequate nutrition and physical activity to help treat this silent bone disease.

## KEY TAKEAWAYS

Non-motor symptoms affect almost all patients living with Parkinson's disease and can have a profound influence on activities of daily living. While nutrition interventions may not be the sole solution for all non-motor symptoms, there are strategies that can help improve symptom management and quality of life.

- Sensory changes, like altered taste and smell, can impact appetite. Focusing on other aspects of meals, such as varying textures, creating a colorful plate and enhancing bold flavors, can help make meals more enjoyable.
- Mood and cognitive challenges, like forgetfulness, anxiety and depression, can change eating habits. Creating low-effort meals, asking for help from friends and family and establishing routines can help ease the burden of meal preparation.
- Constipation can lead to decreased appetite, bloating and abdominal pain. Focusing on fiber, hydration and movement can help promote regular bowel movements.
- Gastroparesis can result in nausea, vomiting and abdominal pain, leading to less optimal nutrition. Focusing on softer, nutrient-dense foods and frequent, small meals can possibly ease these symptoms.
- Nausea and vomiting from gastrointestinal problems or medications can impact the types and amounts of food one is able to consume. Understanding the root cause and focusing on foods that are better tolerated can help ease symptoms.
- Swallowing difficulty can lead to choking and fearfulness when eating. Modifying food textures and adding nutritional supplements can help one meet their nutrition needs with less effort. A feeding tube may be appropriate for some.
- Unintentional weight loss and malnutrition can result from the numerous challenges faced by those living with Parkinson's disease. Understanding the root cause and collaborating with your health-care team is critically important. Focusing on small, nutrient-dense meals and snacks and adding nutritional supplements can help one maintain weight and strength.
- Orthostatic and postprandial hypotension can lead to an increased risk of falls and fractures. Increasing fluid and salt intake can help normalize blood pressure. Avoiding heavy meals and alcohol can be helpful in some cases.
- Osteoporosis can result from poor nutrient intake, less physical activity and the natural aging process. Ensuring adequate calcium, vitamin D and protein intake is essential for bone health. Osteoporosis is twice as common in Parkinson's disease even in men.

## References

Abbott RD, Petrovitch H, White LR, et al. Frequency of bowel movements and the future risk of Parkinson's disease. *Neurology*. 2001 Aug 14;57(3):456-62. doi: 10.1212/wnl.57.3.456. PMID: 11502913.

Academy of Nutrition and Dietetics. Gastroparesis: Nutrition Intervention. Nutrition Care Manual. Accessed November 15, 2025. https://www.nutritioncaremanual.org/topic.cfm?ncm_category_id=1&lv1=5522&lv2=255703&lv3=272814&ncm_toc_id=272814&ncm_heading=Nutrition%20Care.

Academy of Nutrition and Dietetics. Osteoporosis. Nutrition Care Manual. Accessed November 28, 2025. https://www.nutritioncaremanual.org/topic.cfm?ncm_category_id=1&lv1=272978&lv2=21129&lv3=267404&ncm_toc_id=267404&ncm_heading=Nutrition%20Care.

Alia S, Andrenelli E, Di Paolo A, et al. Chemosensory Impairments and Their Impact on Nutrition in Parkinson's Disease: A Narrative Literature Review. Nutrients. 2025 Feb 13;17(4):671. doi: 10.3390/nu17040671. PMID: 40004999; PMCID: PMC11858080.

Carroll C, Clarke CE, Grosset D, et al. Addressing Comorbidities in People with Parkinson's Disease: Considerations From An Expert Panel. *J Parkinsons Dis*. 2024;14(1):53-63. doi: 10.3233/JPD-230168. PMID: 38217610; PMCID: PMC10836549.

Chen B, Yang W, Luo Y, et al. Non-pharmacological and drug treatment of autonomic dysfunction in multiple system atrophy: current status and future directions. *J Neurol*. 2023 Nov;270(11):5251-5273. doi: 10.1007/s00415-023-11876-y. Epub 2023 Jul 21. PMID: 37477834.

Chiang HL, Lin CH. Management of Gastrointestinal Symptoms in Parkinson's Disease. *J Cent Nerv Syst Dis*. 2025 Aug 13;17:11795735251370014. doi: 10.1177/11795735251370014. PMID: 40823476; PMCID: PMC12351107.

Cong S, Xiang C, Zhang S, et al. Prevalence and clinical aspects of depression in Parkinson's disease: A systematic review and metaanalysis of 129 studies. *Neurosci Biobehav Rev*. 2022 Oct;141:104749. doi: 10.1016/j.neubiorev.2022.104749. Epub 2022 Jun 21. PMID: 35750224.

Fanciulli A, Leys F, Falup-Pecurariu C, et al. Management of Orthostatic Hypotension in Parkinson's Disease. *J Parkinsons Dis*. 2020;10(s1):S57-S64. doi: 10.3233/JPD-202036. PMID: 32716319; PMCID: PMC7592655.

Flanagan R, Rusch C, Lithander FE, et al. The missing piece of the puzzle - The key role of the dietitian in the management of Parkinson's disease. *Parkinsonism Relat Disord*. 2024 Apr;121:106021. doi: 10.1016/j.parkreldis.2024.106021. Epub 2024 Feb 1. PMID: 38326170.

International Dysphagia Diet Standardisation Initiative. Level 4 Pureed Food for Adults. 2019 Jan. Accessed December 28, 2025. https://www.iddsi.org/images/Publications-Resources/PatientHandouts/English/Adults/4_pureed_adults_consumer_handout_30jan2019.pdf.

International Dysphagia Diet Standardisation Initiative. Level 5 Minced & Moist Food for Adults. 2019 Jan. Accessed December 28, 2025. https://www.iddsi.org/images/Publications-Resources/PatientHandouts/English/Adults/5_minced_moist_adults_consumer_handout_30jan2019.pdf.

International Dysphagia Diet Standardisation Initiative. Level 6 Soft & Bite Sized for Adults. 2019 Jan. Accessed December 28, 2025. https://www.iddsi.org/images/

Publications-Resources/PatientHandouts/English/Adults/6_soft_bite_sized_adult_consumer_handout_30jan2019.pdf.

International Dysphagia Diet Standardisation Initiative. Level 7 Regular Easy to Chew for Adults. 2019 Jan. Accessed December 28, 2025. https://www.iddsi.org/images/Publications-Resources/PatientHandouts/English/Adults/7_easy_to_chew_adult_consumer_handout_30jan2019.pdf.

Katsirma Z, Dimidi E, Rodriguez-Mateos A, Whelan K. Fruits and their impact on the gut microbiota, gut motility and constipation. *Food Funct.* 2021 Oct 4;12(19):8850-8866. doi: 10.1039/d1fo01125a. PMID: 34505614.

Ó Breasail M, Smith MD, Tenison E, et al. Parkinson's disease: the nutrition perspective. *Proc Nutr Soc.* 2022 Mar;81(1):12-26. doi: 10.1017/S0029665121003645. Epub 2021 Oct 4. Erratum in: Proc Nutr Soc. 2023 Dec;82(4):487. doi: 10.1017/S0029665122000787. PMID: 35105409.

Schindler A, Pizzorni N, Cereda E, et al. Consensus on the treatment of dysphagia in Parkinson's disease. *J Neurol Sci.* 2021 Nov 15;430:120008. doi: 10.1016/j.jns.2021.120008. Epub 2021 Sep 27. PMID: 34624796.

Soliman H, Coffin B, Gourcerol G. Gastroparesis in Parkinson Disease: Pathophysiology, and Clinical Management. Brain Sci. 2021 Jun 23;11(7):831. doi: 10.3390/brainsci11070831. PMID: 34201699; PMCID: PMC8301889.

U.S. Department of Agriculture and U.S. Department of Health and Human Services. Dietary Guidelines for Americans, 2020-2025. 9th ed. 2020. Accessed November 29, 2025. https://www.dietaryguidelines.gov/sites/default/files/2021-03/Dietary_Guidelines_for_Americans-2020-2025.pdf.

U.S. Department of Health and Human Services. Calcium Fact Sheet for Health Professionals. National Institutes of Health Office of Dietary Supplements. Updated July 11, 2025. Accessed November 28, 2025. https://ods.od.nih.gov/factsheets/Calcium-HealthProfessional/.

U.S. Department of Health and Human Services. Vitamin D Fact Sheet for Health Professionals. National Institutes of Health Office of Dietary Supplements. Updated June 27, 2025. Accessed November 28, 2025. https://ods.od.nih.gov/factsheets/VitaminD-HealthProfessional/.

U.S. Department of Health and Human Services. Zinc Fact Sheet for Health Professionals. National Institutes of Health Office of Dietary Supplements. Updated September 28, 2022. Accessed November 28, 2025. https://ods.od.nih.gov/factsheets/zinc-healthprofessional/.

Vloet LC, Mehagnoul-Schipper DJ, Hoefnagels WH, et al. The influence of low-, normal-, and high-carbohydrate meals on blood pressure in elderly patients with postprandial hypotension. *J Gerontol A Biol Sci Med Sci.* 2001 Dec;56(12):M744-8. doi: 10.1093/gerona/56.12.m744. PMID: 11723147.

White JV, Guenter P, Jensen G, et al; Academy of Nutrition and Dietetics Malnutrition Work Group; A.S.P.E.N. Malnutrition Task Force; A.S.P.E.N. Board of Directors. Consensus statement of the Academy of Nutrition and Dietetics/American Society for Parenteral and Enteral Nutrition: characteristics recommended for the identification and documentation of adult malnutrition (undernutrition). *J Acad Nutr Diet.* 2012 May;112(5):730-8. doi: 10.1016/j.jand.2012.03.012. Epub 2012 Apr 25. Erratum in: J Acad Nutr Diet. 2012 Nov;112(11):1899. Erratum in: J Acad Nutr Diet. 2017 Mar;117(3):480. doi: 10.1016/j.jand.2017.01.021. PMID: 22709779.

## CHAPTER 5

# DIET–MEDICATION INTERACTIONS

*The common challenges with diet and medications include meal and medication timing and avoidance of specific nutrients.*

Medications prescribed to help manage Parkinson's disease symptoms can have various interactions with many foods. These interactions not only affect the way the medications are absorbed and how well they work, but they can also affect a person's nutritional status. The common challenges with diet and medications include meal and medication timing and avoidance of specific nutrients. Understanding how medications can interact with the diet can help to avoid fluctuations in symptom management and can in some cases lead to a reduction in side effects. This section outlines key medication–nutrient interactions. Much more research is needed on other potential medication interactions, so be sure to talk to a health-care professional for the latest guidance in your specific case.

## Carbidopa-Levodopa

Carbidopa-levodopa is a medication used to treat motor symptoms in people living with Parkinson's disease. It works by replacing lost dopamine. The levodopa portion of the medication is converted to dopamine in the brain. The carbidopa portion of the medication prevents the levodopa from converting to dopamine before the medication reaches the brain, and it is known to reduce nausea.

While intended to improve motor symptoms, levodopa therapy is associated with changes in symptoms especially as Parkinson's disease progresses. Some patients on levodopa therapy experience wearing off or shorter response times. Others might experience an on-off phenomenon, which manifests as fluctuations in motor symptoms. Even with carbidopa helping the dopamine to reach the brain, it's estimated that only a small percentage of levodopa crosses the force field called the blood-brain barrier. This translates to less dopamine being supplied to the brain to help reduce a person's motor symptoms.

Because levodopa therapy is not a one-size-fits-all treatment, it is important to create individualized plans to maximize how much levodopa gets to the brain. There are many factors that can interfere with how the medication is being used, including dietary patterns and gastrointestinal problems (discussed in Chapter 4).

### Dietary Protein and Levodopa

High protein diets may interfere with levodopa absorption and lead to motor symptom fluctuations. This happens because amino acids, which are the building blocks of proteins in the diet, and levodopa use the same transport system. Both amino acids and levodopa are competing to be picked up by the same transporters that were made to move amino acids into the brain. Therefore, if levodopa enters the body at the same time as a protein-rich meal, the transporters may pick up the amino acids instead of the levodopa.

While this interaction can be a problem and efforts should be made to maximize the efficacy of levodopa, this fight for transporters does not appear to be an issue for most people. A study of 877 participants showed that only 5.9%, or 6 out of 100 people, reported an interaction between levodopa and protein in their diets. For most people, taking carbidopa-levodopa on an empty stomach (about 30 minutes before a meal or 1 to 2 hours after a meal) minimizes the potential for interaction.

While uncommon and typically observed only in moderate to advanced stages of Parkinson's disease, there are strategies to minimize levodopa and dietary protein interactions for those who experience motor fluctuations associated with dietary protein consumption. These strategies include limiting the amount of protein in the diet, as well as timing protein consumption around medications.

### LEVODOPA AND FOOD BALANCE

- Levodopa competes with amino acids (protein building blocks).
- Take levodopa about 30 minutes before meals if possible.
- Consider shifting protein intake to later in the day if symptoms fluctuate.
- Do not eliminate protein as balance and timing are key.
- Track your response and adjust with your care team.

### LOW-PROTEIN DIET

A limited number of studies have revealed that a low-protein diet could stabilize the effects of levodopa. However, the definition for a low-protein diet has not been well-established. It is thought that a low-protein diet contains less than the recommended daily allowance (RDA) of protein (<0.8g/kg body weight/day). High-quality studies on low-protein diets and levodopa efficacy are lacking, meaning there is not enough evidence to state that a low-protein diet is an evidence-based option. In fact, a low-protein diet is likely not sustainable as it could lead to nutritional deficiencies and increase one's risk for malnutrition. Currently, a low-protein diet is not recommended due to the lack of supporting evidence.

### PROTEIN-REDISTRIBUTION DIET

A protein-redistribution diet involves redistributing protein needs throughout the day. Typically, one limits the amount of protein consumed at breakfast and lunch and eats larger amounts of protein in the evening. This diet limits interactions during the day when medication fluctuations are more likely to interfere with activities of daily living. Protein-redistribution diets are better understood when compared to low-protein diets. A protein-redistribution diet is associated with improvement in motor symptoms and lower disability scores. Protein-redistribution diets are more sustainable, meaning they are more feasible to adhere to for a longer period. When using this diet strategy, the risk of levodopa-induced dyskinesias may increase, and medication adjustments may be necessary in collaboration with your health-care provider. Weight should also be monitored as changes in protein consumption may lead to unintentional weight loss.

| REGULAR DIET | PROTEIN-REDISTRIBUTION DIET |
|---|---|
| For an individual with a daily protein goal of 70-80 grams | |
| **BREAKFAST**<br>• 2 eggs (12 g protein)<br>• 1 slice whole wheat toast with peanut butter (8 g protein)<br>• ½ cup (125 mL) strawberries<br>**LUNCH**<br>• 3 oz (90 g) grilled chicken breast (26 g protein)<br>• ½ cup (125 mL) cooked quinoa (4 g protein)<br>• 1 cup (250 mL) mixed vegetables<br>**SNACK**<br>• Low-fat cottage cheese with pineapple chunks (14 g protein)<br>**DINNER**<br>• 2 black bean tacos with shredded cheese (15 g protein)<br>• Vegetable toppings | **BREAKFAST**<br>• 1 egg (6 g protein)<br>• 1 slice whole wheat toast (4 g protein)<br>• ½ cup (125 mL) strawberries<br>**SNACK**<br>• 2 tbsp (30 mL) almonds (4 g protein)<br>• Dried fruit<br>**LUNCH**<br>• Hummus wrap with vegetables and feta cheese (10 g protein)<br>**SNACK**<br>• Cheese and crackers (5 g protein)<br>**DINNER**<br>• 6 oz (175 mL) grilled chicken breast (38 g protein)<br>• ½ cup (125 mL) cooked quinoa (4 g protein)<br>• Vegetables |
| Total Protein: 79 grams | Total Protein: 71 grams |

### Other Meal Components and Levodopa

Some people taking levodopa might experience fluctuations in symptom relief associated with all forms of eating, not just with high-protein meals. This phenomenon may be explained by the nutrient content. Meals that are high in fat and/or fiber take longer for the stomach to digest. If levodopa is taken close to a meal that is high in either of these nutrients, it may take longer to be absorbed as it mixes with the meal contents already present in the stomach. This is especially true for people who experience delayed gastric emptying (see Chapter 4). If there is a delay in levodopa absorption, there is likely to be a delay in symptom relief. People who experience this interaction should be careful to limit the fat and fiber content of meals and/or time medications so they are taken far apart from mealtimes.

## COMMON SOURCES OF MEALTIME FATS

- Butters and oils
- Creamy sauces, condiments and gravies
- High-fat dairy (whole milk, cheese, yogurt, heavy cream)
- Fried foods
- Red and processed meats
- Fatty fish, avocados, nuts and seeds*

*Fatty fish, avocados, nuts and seeds can be beneficial for brain health and should be a part of a balanced diet. However, people that find their medications do not work well in close proximity to high-fat meals should limit their intake of these foods close to when they take their medications.

## COMMON SOURCES OF MEALTIME FIBER*

- Whole grains (whole wheat bread, whole wheat pasta, brown rice, etc.)
- Vegetables (leafy greens, potatoes, broccoli, etc.)
- Legumes (nuts, beans, peas, etc.)
- Fruits

*Fiber is an important part of a balanced diet and should not be excluded. However, people that find their medications do not work well in close proximity to high-fiber meals should limit the amount of fiber they consume close to when they take their medications.

## Monoamine Oxidase Inhibitors (MAO-Is)

A monoamine oxidase inhibitor (MAO-I) is a medication that stops the enzyme monoamine oxidase. An enzyme is a helper protein in your body that makes chemical reactions happen faster and more efficiently. It acts like a key or a tool, helping molecules fit together or break apart without being used up. Without enzymes, many of the processes that keep you alive, like digestion, energy production and brain signaling, would happen far too slowly. There are different types of MAOs and MAO-Is that can be used to inhibit enzymes. Monoamine oxidase B (MAO-B) metabolizes or breaks down dopamine, which can decrease the amount of time that levodopa works, leading to more "off" medication times. Some patients are prescribed MAO-B inhibitors to improve levodopa effectiveness. Common MAO-B inhibitors include selegiline, rasagiline and safinamide. MAO-Is can also be used to treat depression. In Parkinson's disease we use only MAO-B inhibitors and we do so at low dosage. Higher dosages can also activate MAO-A receptors in the brain and result in what is known as the cheese effect.

### BALANCING INHIBITORS

- Medications like carbidopa, MAO-B inhibitors, and COMT inhibitors help dopamine "on" periods last longer.
- These inhibitors prevent breakdown of dopamine or levodopa.
- Balance is critical to avoid side effects like dyskinesia.
- Medication plans should be personalized and adjusted over time.
- If taking a MAO-B type inhibitor, changes to the diet should only be made if you are taking higher doses. Otherwise, tyramine-containing foods are safe to eat.

### Tyramine, MAO-Is and the Cheese Effect

One type of MAO degrades a compound called tyramine, which is naturally found in many foods. It is found in higher amounts in aged and fermented foods, such as aged cheese, yogurt and red wine. Tyramine is degraded specifically by type A MAOs. When a MAO-A inhibitor is present, this prevents the degradation of tyramine. In response, tyramine is taken up by brain cells, which can lead to hypertensive crisis or critically high blood pressure. For this reason, people taking MAO-A inhibitors should follow a tyramine-restricted diet.

Since a diet–medication interaction is typically seen with MAO-A inhibitors, not everyone taking a MAO-B inhibitor should follow a tyramine-restricted diet. However, at higher doses, MAO-B inhibitors may also bind to type A MAOs, leading to less degradation of tyramine. If higher doses of MAO-B inhibitors in tablet form are required, your dietitian might advise you to limit the number and overall amount of tyramine-containing foods you consume.

## WHAT DIET SHOULD I FOLLOW IF I TAKE AN MAO-B INHIBITOR?

A tyramine-restricted diet may be recommended only if you take high doses of MAO-B inhibitors. Talk to your neurologist and/or registered dietitian if you take higher doses of selegiline (>10 mg/day) or rasagiline (>2 mg/day). Safinamide is least likely to interact with tyramine. Most Parkinson's experts do not prescribe high-dose MAO-B drugs and thus the cheese effect should not be a worry.

## TYRAMINE-RESTRICTED DIET

A tyramine-restricted diet limits the consumption of foods with high amounts of tyramine.

**Foods to Avoid**

- Fermented vegetables (e.g., sauerkraut, kimchi)
- Fermented or spoiled fruit
- Aged cheese (e.g., Cheddar, Gouda, Muenster, feta)
- Fermented meat products (e.g., chorizo, salchichon)
- Corned beef and imported pepperoni
- Meat products near or beyond their expiration date
- Wine and beer
- Fermented soy products (e.g., soy sauce, soybean curd)
- Yeast extracts

**Recommended Foods**

- Fresh, frozen or canned fruits and vegetables
- Milk, and processed cheese made from pasteurized milk
- Fresh cheese (e.g., cottage cheese, ricotta)
- Fresh meat and fish
- Ham and smoked meats
- Pepperoni products in the United States

## References

Academy of Nutrition and Dietetics. Tyramine-restricted nutrition therapy. Nutrition Care Manual. Accessed August 28, 2025. https://www.nutritioncaremanual.org/client_ed.cfm?ncm_client_ed_id=12.

Agnieszka W, Paweł P, Małgorzata K. How to Optimize the Effectiveness and Safety of Parkinson's Disease Therapy? - A Systematic Review of Drugs Interactions with Food and Dietary Supplements. *Curr Neuropharmacol.* 2022;20(7):1427-1447. doi: 10.2174/1570159X19666211116142806. PMID: 34784871; PMCID: PMC9881082.

Boelens Keun JT, Arnoldussen IA, Vriend C, et al. Dietary Approaches to Improve Efficacy and Control Side Effects of Levodopa Therapy in Parkinson's Disease: A Systematic Review. *Adv Nutr.* 2021 Dec 1;12(6):2265-2287. doi: 10.1093/advances/nmab060. PMID: 34113965; PMCID: PMC8634393.

Rusch C, Flanagan R, Suh H, et al. To restrict or not to restrict? Practical considerations for optimizing dietary protein interactions on levodopa absorption in Parkinson's disease. *NPJ Parkinsons Dis.* 2023 Jun 24;9(1):98. doi: 10.1038/s41531-023-00541-w. PMID: 37355689; PMCID: PMC10290638.

# CHAPTER 6

# A LETTER TO PARKINSON'S CARE PARTNERS ON NUTRITION

## Dear care partner,

If you are reading this, you are likely carrying a great deal of responsibility and love. Nutrition may seem like a small piece of the Parkinson's disease puzzle; however, it is one of the few areas where daily choices can meaningfully influence energy, thinking, mood, gut health and overall quality of life. You are not expected to be perfect. You are asked to be attentive, flexible and kind to yourself and to the person you love.

Parkinson's disease changes how the body moves, digests and responds to food. Appetite can fluctuate. Swallowing can become effortful. Constipation may dominate daily life. Medications may compete with protein for gut absorption. Your role is not to enforce rules, but rather to help create balance.

Below is a practical framework to guide you:

### Prioritize regular meals

Skipping meals worsens fatigue, dizziness and medication side effects. Help establish consistent mealtimes even when appetite is low.

### Be strategic about protein

Protein is essential for muscle and strength; however, it can interfere with levodopa absorption for some. Some folks do better when most protein is shifted to the evening meal rather than breakfast or lunch. In rare cases where protein is impeding the absorption of Parkinson's medications, give the medications a half an hour head start before eating.

**Support the gut**

Constipation affects most folks with Parkinson's and can worsen many of the symptoms. Encourage fiber-rich foods such as vegetables, fruits, beans and whole grains along with adequate fluids spread throughout the day.

**Hydration matters more than you think**

Dehydration contributes to confusion, low blood pressure, falls and constipation. Gentle reminders and visible water access can make a real difference. Six to eight glasses of water per day is optimal.

**Simplify food choices**

Fatigue and slowness can transform meals into an overwhelming experience. Simple, nutrient-dense foods prepared ahead of time can reduce stress and improve consistency.

**Watch for weight changes**

Unintentional weight loss is common and often missed. Regular "weigh-ins" allow early course correction before strength and resilience are lost.

**Adapt for swallowing safety**

If coughing, choking or food-sticking appear, involve speech and swallow specialists early. Texture adjustments can preserve nutrition and prevent pneumonia. A speech language pathologist along with a dietitian can individualize a plan to enhance swallowing safety and to preserve quality of life.

**Respect pleasure and culture**
Food is more than fuel. It is connection, memory and joy. Make room for favorite foods and shared meals whenever possible.

**Avoid extreme diets**
There is no single Parkinson's diet. Be cautious with restrictive plans that promise cures. Balance is usually a better approach than following an extreme diet.

**Ask for help**
Dietitians, speech therapists and health-care providers can individualize guidance. You do not have to solve this alone.

## A Final Word

You are doing important work. Small daily adjustments add up over time. When nutrition improves, energy improves. When energy improves, movement, thinking and mood frequently follow. Progress may be uneven; however, your steady presence matters more than perfection.

Care partners change outcomes. Your attention at the table echoes far beyond the meal.

PART III

# DIET CONSIDERATIONS FOR PARKINSON'S DISEASE

CHAPTER 7

# POPULAR AND UNPOPULAR DIETS

*Diet matters because it is becoming increasingly evident that nutrition could be a modifiable risk factor for the later development of Parkinson's disease.*

The term "diet" is commonly used in everyday conversation as a reference to food choices aligning with a person's ideal image of being healthy. Diet actually refers to habitual eating patterns, whether healthy or not. Diet matters because it is becoming increasingly evident that nutrition could be a modifiable risk factor for the later development of Parkinson's disease. For those already living with Parkinson's, diet may serve as an avenue for targeted therapy for managing symptoms and possibly one day for slowing disease progression.

Several studies suggest a connection between diet and disease progression. There are also studies revealing the importance of diet on symptom management. Processes such as oxidative stress, neuroinflammation and alterations in the gut microbiome may be at play when choosing a diet for Parkinson's disease:

- Dietary antioxidants, such as vitamins C and E, are thought to act as neuroprotective factors against oxidative stress and loss of brain cells. Several studies have shown a connection between higher antioxidant consumption and a lower risk for the later development of Parkinson's disease.
- High-fiber diets have been associated with increased short-chain fatty acid (SCFA) production, a potentially important factor for maintaining the integrity of the blood-brain barrier and for preventing neuroinflammation.
- Diets high in fermentable fiber support a diverse gut microbiome and can help maintain bowel regularity.

Rather than focusing on individual nutrients, overall dietary patterns can be used to capture an array of beneficial food components. For this reason, this chapter will focus on diet patterns that have been studied in Parkinson's disease. Each section will highlight beneficial components, as well as the potential risks or pitfalls with following each diet.

## Gluten-Free Diet

A gluten-free diet, like the name suggests, eliminates foods that contain gluten. Gluten, a protein naturally found in certain grains, helps provide structure to foods like bread, pasta, cereals and baked goods. It can also be found in sauces (e.g., soy sauce), salad dressings, gravies, Brewer's yeast, beer and malt products that are derived from gluten-containing grains. Other grains that are naturally gluten-free, like oats, may be exposed to gluten in manufacturing facilities that also process gluten-containing grains.

### GLUTEN-CONTAINING GRAINS

- Wheat
- Barley
- Rye
- Triticale
- Oats (unless packaging indicates they are gluten-free)

### GLUTEN-FREE GRAINS

- Amaranth
- Arrowroot
- Buckwheat
- Cassava (manioc)
- Corn
- Flax
- Indian rice grass
- Job's tears
- Millet and finger millet (ragi)
- Quinoa
- Rice
- Sago
- Sorghum
- Tapioca
- Teff
- Wild rice
- Yucca

Gluten has known adverse effects on individuals living with gluten allergies, celiac disease and gluten sensitivities:

- People living with a *gluten allergy* experience an immunologic reaction minutes to hours after gluten exposure. A wide range of symptoms might occur, including itching, swelling, abdominal pain, nausea, diarrhea, headache, wheezing and shortness of breath. Diagnosing a gluten allergy involves lab tests that identify antibodies to gluten.

- People living with *celiac disease* experience an autoimmune reaction that develops over weeks to years in response to gluten exposure. Symptoms might include diarrhea, abdominal pain, anemia, osteoporosis and neurological symptoms. Genetic factors may also play a role in celiac disease, and a diagnosis can sometimes be made by looking at specific biomarkers or gene tests.
- People living with a *gluten sensitivity* experience an immune-mediated response hours to days after gluten exposure. Symptoms might include abdominal pain, diarrhea, weight loss, bloating and fatigue. Since there are no biomarkers to diagnose gluten sensitivity, clinicians must rely on clinical presentation and the exclusion of a gluten allergy or the presence of celiac disease.

The current data suggests 1% to 2% of the general population is living with celiac disease and that 1% to 13% of the general population is living with gluten sensitivity. For each condition, a gluten-free diet may mediate the symptoms.

While the role of gluten in celiac disease and gluten sensitivities is known, research on how gluten consumption affects people living with Parkinson's disease has been limited. Some studies suggest a link between gluten sensitivities and an increased risk for Parkinson's disease. Researchers believe that gluten consumption could cause a chronic inflammatory state in the GI tract that may in some cases spread to include systemic inflammation throughout the entire body. For people with celiac disease, gluten consumption is known to damage the intestinal lining. A damaged intestinal lining allows microbes to exit the GI tract and to travel to other body systems. While gluten itself does not cause Parkinson's disease, its potential to induce neuroinflammation could possibly influence disease onset and progression. For gluten-sensitive individuals, reducing gluten consumption may be beneficial.

On the other hand, some studies show no significant association between gluten consumption and Parkinson's disease. More research will be needed to understand how a gluten-containing diet might affect people living with Parkinson's disease and whether this is a beneficial strategy.

People following a gluten-free diet should be careful to ensure they do not eliminate important nutrients. Gluten-free diets could lack enough carbohydrates, fiber, vitamins

### UNDERSTANDING THE EFFECTS OF GLUTEN

#### GLUTEN ALLERGY

- Allergic reaction to gluten
- Minutes to hours after gluten exposure
- Symptoms include itching, swelling, abdominal pain, GI discomfort, etc.
- Diagnosed through lab tests to identify antibodies

#### CELIAC DISEASE

- Autoimmune response to gluten exposure
- Develops over weeks to years
- Symptoms include diarrhea, abdominal pain, anemia, osteoporosis, and neurological symptoms
- Diagnosed through clinic presentation, biomarkers, or genetic factors

#### GLUTEN SENSITIVITY

- Immune-mediated response to gluten (not as severe as an allergy)
- Hours to days after gluten exposure
- Symptoms include abdominal pain, weight loss, diarrhea, fatigue, etc.
- Diagnosed through exclusion of gluten allergy and celiac disease

and minerals. Specifically, this diet is low in folate, niacin, vitamin D, vitamin $B_{12}$, iron, calcium, phosphorus and zinc. It is essential to replace gluten-containing grains with gluten-free grains in order to more fully meet nutrient requirements.

### GLUTEN-FREE DIET CONCLUSIONS

People living with celiac disease or those who have a known gluten sensitivity should follow a gluten-free diet. There is not enough evidence to recommend a gluten-free diet for people living with Parkinson's disease in the absence of a gluten allergy or gluten sensitivity. A gluten-free diet is safe to follow; however, people should make efforts to replace gluten-containing grains with gluten-free grains so as to not eliminate important fiber, vitamins and minerals.

## Ketogenic Diet

The ketogenic (keto) diet is an eating pattern that limits carbohydrate intake and emphasizes foods high in fat. It typically restricts carbohydrate intake to less than 50 grams per day to as low as 20 grams per day. The diet is designed to shift the body's main fuel source from glucose, which is obtained from carbohydrates, to ketones. Ketones are produced in periods of starvation, fasting and exercise and can be used as an energy source in the absence of enough glucose. This survival mechanism is termed ketogenesis.

**TYPICAL KETOGENIC DIET RATIOS**

| FAT | PROTEIN | CARBOHYDRATES |
|---|---|---|
| 70%–80% of total daily calories | 10%–20% of total daily calories | 5%–10% of total daily calories |

### WHAT ARE CARBOHYDRATES?

When consumed, carbohydrates are broken down into glucose molecules, which are the body's main source of energy. Carbohydrates are found in grains, starchy vegetables, fruits and products with higher amounts of sugar. Common examples include bread, pasta, rice, potatoes, corn, beans, legumes, fruit, fruit juice and other sugary beverages, as well as candy and dessert items.

The keto diet is primarily recommended for individuals who have epilepsy; however, it has gained more attention recently in neurodegenerative diseases for its ability to reduce inflammation and to aid in brain cell energy production. While there are many potential ways it could benefit people living with Parkinson's disease, it has not been heavily researched. Most studies have been of short duration, include a small number of participants and do not follow the same protocols, meaning we cannot draw conclusions about how the diet might benefit most people living with Parkinson's disease. Of the limited studies, improvements have been observed in non-motor symptoms, including fatigue, pain and cognitive impairment. One study showed improvements in exercise endurance.

When considering a ketogenic diet, it is important to understand the side effects. The ketogenic diet may lead to weight loss, which may be beneficial for some. However, people living with Parkinson's disease who are already at an appropriate weight may experience unintentional weight loss that is harder to control and could lead to further health consequences (see Chapter 4). It is better in Parkinson's disease to be a little heavier than a little lighter in weight, as weight loss occurs in almost all cases. Other side effects include hunger, fatigue, mood swings, constipation and headaches. Nutrient deficiencies are a concern with any restrictive diet. In this case, for example, not eating enough grains could lead to less intake of B vitamins, which are essential for people living with Parkinson's disease. Additionally, following a ketogenic diet in the long term has been associated with an increased risk for kidney stones and osteoporosis.

## KETOGENIC DIET CONCLUSIONS

While preliminary evidence is promising, more research is needed to understand how the ketogenic diet might improve Parkinson's symptoms in the long term. This diet could lead to unintentional weight loss, fatigue, mood swings, constipation, headaches and nutrient deficiencies. Given the limited amount of research and potential for adverse health outcomes, currently a ketogenic diet is not generally recommended for people living with Parkinson's disease.

## Mediterranean Diet

The Mediterranean diet is an eating pattern that was inspired by cuisine from countries in the region of the Mediterranean Sea. The Mediterranean diet is largely a plant-based approach that emphasizes fruits, vegetables, whole grains, fish, nuts, seeds and olive oil. Poultry, eggs and dairy products are included in moderate amounts, and red meats and ultra-processed foods are limited. Other components of the Mediterranean diet include opting for whole grains, consuming wine with meals and choosing low-fat dairy products. Additionally, cooking with herbs and spices is also recommended if following this diet. Rather than restricting entire foods or food groups, the Mediterranean diet promotes moderation and long-term sustainability. This diet also encourages shared meals and regular physical activity.

The Mediterranean diet is promoted for better management of cardiovascular disease, diabetes, metabolic syndrome, gastrointestinal conditions and other chronic diseases, including Parkinson's. Because inflammation, oxidative stress and gut dysfunction are all implicated in Parkinson's disease, this eating pattern is frequently used for its potential anti-inflammatory and antioxidant-rich qualities. Many Mediterranean diet staples, including fruits, vegetables, olive oil and fish, all contain compounds that may help to reduce oxidative stress and support heart and brain health.

- The Mediterranean diet is high in **fiber** derived from fruits, vegetables, whole grains and legumes. Fiber is important for gut health, satiety and energy regulation.
- The Mediterranean diet promotes the consumption of **unsaturated fats** from olive oil, avocados and fatty fish. These healthy fats help to reduce inflammation and can be important for the health of your brain cells.
- The Mediterranean diet is high in **antioxidants**, which come from colorful fruits and vegetables, spices and red wine. Antioxidants help to reduce oxidative stress.
- The Mediterranean diet contains a variety of **vitamins and minerals** from whole foods, including fruits, vegetables and whole grains. Vitamins and minerals are important for supporting brain and body cell functions, bone health and energy.

### MEDITERRANEAN DIET BENEFITS

- Supports brain and heart health
- Rich in fruits, vegetables, whole grains
- Includes healthy fats (olive oil, fish)
- Associated with better cognitive outcomes
- Supports gut microbiome
- Anti-inflammatory pattern
- Reduces oxidative stress

## MEDITERRANEAN DIET COMPONENTS

| FOODS TO EAT | |
|---|---|
| Vegetables | ≥2 servings daily |
| Fruits, including 100% fruit juice | ≥3 serving daily |
| Legumes | ≥3 servings weekly |
| Olive oil | ≥4 tablespoons (¼ cup) daily |
| Fish or seafood | ≥3 servings weekly |
| Poultry, eggs and dairy | "Moderate" consumption |
| Sofrito* | ≥2 servings weekly |
| Herbs and spices | Specific amount not established |
| **FOODS TO LIMIT** | |
| Sweets (added sugars) | <1 sugar-sweetened beverage daily<br><3 servings commercial sweets or pastries that are not homemade weekly |
| Red meats or processed meat products | <1 serving daily |
| Butter, margarine or cream | <1 serving daily |
| **ALCOHOL RECOMMENDATIONS** | |
| Wine | ≥7 glasses weekly (see #9 in list on page 90) |

*Sofrito is a sauce made with tomatoes, onion, garlic and olive oil. It can be served with vegetables, pasta, rice and other dishes.

## TIPS FOR FOLLOWING A MEDITERRANEAN-STYLE DIET

1. Use olive oil abundantly for dressings and cooking. Limit solid fat sources, like butter, margarine and lard.
2. Include a variety of fruits and vegetables, aiming for at least 5 servings of produce per day.
3. Include nuts and seeds, which can be added to salads, smoothies and cereals.
4. Eat legumes, like beans and lentils, which are great sources of protein, fiber, vitamins and minerals.
5. Choose 100% whole-grain for breads, pastas, cereals and rice.
6. Consume fish weekly. Focus on fatty fish, like salmon, tuna, mackerel or sardines.
7. Choose low-fat dairy products over full-fat dairy.
8. Limit red meat consumption and opt for leaner meats, like poultry without the skin. Limit packaged meats, like hot dogs, luncheon meats and sausages.
9. For usual drinkers, include a glass of wine with meals. Limit consumption to 5 oz (150 mL) per day for women and 10 oz (300 mL) per day for men. Wine may need to be limited in Parkinson's especially if gait and balance dysfunction are present.
10. Limit concentrated sources of sugar, including sugar-sweetened beverages and dessert items.
11. Limit fried foods, and try to eat home-cooked meals.
12. Aim for 8 cups (2 L) of water per day or an appropriate amount as directed by your health-care team.

Most evidence on the Mediterranean diet for Parkinson's disease has been provided from observational studies, meaning that the many findings are based solely on observing people who follow a Mediterranean-style diet. While researchers have tried to eliminate other variables that could influence the results of their studies, this study format has not enabled researchers to conclude that the observed diet alone is what changes outcomes in Parkinson's. Nevertheless, following this diet pattern has been associated with a lower risk of developing Parkinson's disease, and ongoing research has been examining whether this diet pattern could slow the progression of the disease possibly through its impacts on the gut-brain axis. While the findings are still limited, some studies have revealed a possible slower progression of symptoms in people already diagnosed with Parkinson's disease. There are many ways that the Mediterranean diet might impact the disease course:

1. Research shows a portion of people living with Parkinson's disease have an imbalance of bacteria in the gut, termed dysbiosis. This means the gut has an overgrowth of bad bacteria and less of the good bacteria. Dysbiosis can compromise the strength of the intestinal barrier, allowing harmful, inflammatory microbes to escape. The Mediterranean diet's high-fiber content feeds beneficial bacteria in the gut, leading to a better-balanced gut microbiome. This diet promotes moderation and encourages consuming a variety of food groups, which is important for providing an array of vitamins and minerals to support a diverse ecosystem for the gut. The high-polyphenol content of the Mediterranean diet also helps balance the microbiome. Polyphenols are chemical compounds found in olive oil, berries, herbs, spices and legumes, and they are metabolized by gut bacteria to promote the growth of beneficial microbes. Polyphenols may also help lower the concentration of harmful bacteria.
2. Not only does the Mediterranean diet fuel beneficial gut bacteria, but it also helps promote regular bowel movements. Constipation is one of the most common non-motor symptoms of Parkinson's disease, and it can impact how non-parkinsonian medications work and impact quality of life. The Mediterranean diet, high in fiber, is associated with an improvement in constipation symptoms. The Mediterranean diet may positively impact the time it takes for stool to move through the intestine, which further supports a balanced gut microbiome. Prolonged intestinal transit time has been associated with an imbalance in gut bacteria.
3. The Mediterranean diet might also support the integrity of the intestinal barrier, leading to less inflammation. High in fiber, antioxidants and polyphenols, the Mediterranean diet supports short-chain fatty acid (SCFA) production. SCFAs are important for energy balance, immune response and blood-brain barrier strength. However, a decrease in the amount of SCFAs has been observed in the guts of people living with Parkinson's disease. Without enough SCFAs, the intestinal barrier becomes inflamed and may allow harmful microbes to escape. Research

has revealed that there are beneficial effects of the Mediterranean diet on the production of SCFAs in people with Parkinson's disease. A more diverse microbiome is important for maintaining the strength of the intestinal barrier. As previously mentioned, many components of the Mediterranean diet support a well-balanced gut microbiome.

4. The anti-inflammatory components of the Mediterranean diet may also play a role in the course of Parkinson's disease. Foods high in unsaturated fats, including fatty fish, olive oil, nuts and seeds, may help to reduce inflammation. The Mediterranean diet also recommends limiting pro-inflammatory components, like saturated fats, concentrated sweets and ultra-processed foods. A diet high in anti-inflammatory foods and low in pro-inflammatory foods could play a role in reducing intestinal and systemic inflammation. Supporting gut barrier function, reducing inflammation and improving microbial balance may be the keys for the Mediterranean diet in influencing processes linked to α-synuclein misfolding and to neuroinflammation. More research will hopefully enlighten us as to why so many studies in Parkinson's disease suggest a Mediterranean diet is beneficial.

## PROPOSED ROLE OF THE GUT-BRAIN AXIS IN PARKINSON'S DISEASE

1. An imbalance of gut bacteria leads to an immune response (inflammation) in the gut.
2. Inflammation in the gut weakens the intestinal lining, allowing microbes and inflammatory molecules to leave the gut.
3. This immune response spreads to other areas of the body, causing systemic inflammation.
4. The immune system responds to areas of the brain (neuroinflammation), possibly triggering misfolding of α-syn proteins.

## HOW THE MEDITERRANEAN DIET INFLUENCES THE GUT-BRAIN AXIS IN PARKINSON'S DISEASE

- The Mediterranean diet includes key sources of fermentable fiber. Fiber is the primary fuel source for beneficial gut bacteria. A diet high in fiber supports a diverse gut microbiome and regular bowel movements. This is especially important for people living with Parkinson's disease as constipation and an imbalance of gut bacteria (overgrowth of bad bacteria) are common.
- The Mediterranean diet, high in fiber, antioxidants and polyphenols, supports short-chain fatty acid (SCFA) production. SCFAs are important for energy balance, immune response and blood-brain barrier integrity; however, a decrease in the number of SCFAs has been observed in the guts of people living with Parkinson's disease. Following a Mediterranean diet increases SCFA concentration and leads to less intestinal inflammation.
- The Mediterranean diet embraces moderation and supports diverse food choices. Food diversity feeds an ecosystem of bacteria in the gut, which is linked to better gut resilience and reduced inflammation. Since gut dysbiosis (an imbalance of gut bacteria) is linked to Parkinson's disease, supporting bacterial diversity may be an important key.
- The Mediterranean diet includes anti-inflammatory foods, like fatty fish, olive oil, nuts and seeds. It also recommends limiting pro-inflammatory components, like saturated fats, concentrated sweets and ultra-processed foods. A diet high in anti-inflammatory foods and low in pro-inflammatory foods could play a role in reducing neuroinflammation.
- The Mediterranean diet is high in polyphenols, compounds found in olive oil, berries, herbs, spices and legumes. Polyphenols are metabolized by gut bacteria to promote the growth of beneficial microbes and they may lower the concentration of harmful bacteria.
- Following a Mediterranean diet is associated with a reduction in constipation symptoms. The high fiber content of the Mediterranean diet supports gut motility. This is especially important in Parkinson's disease as prolonged gut transit time is common and can lead to imbalances in the gut microbiome.
- While direct evidence is limited, by supporting gut barrier function, reducing inflammation and improving microbial balance, the Mediterranean diet may indirectly influence processes linked to $\alpha$-synuclein misfolding and neuroinflammation.

## How well do you adhere to the Mediterranean diet?

**Instructions**

1. Write your answer to the following 14 questions in the "Answer" column.
2. Use the MEDAS scoring instructions below to score your answers in the "Points" column.
3. Add up your points and use the Score Interpretation guide to see how well you adhere to the Mediterranean diet.

| MEDITERRANEAN DIET ADHERENCE SCREENER (MEDAS) | ANSWER | POINTS |
|---|---|---|
| **1. Do you use olive oil as your main cooking fat?** | | |
| **2. How many tablespoons of olive oil do you use each day?**<br>Include olive oil used in salads, meals eaten away from home and frying. (One tablespoon equals 15 mL.) | | |
| **3. How many servings of vegetables do you eat per day?**<br>One serving = ½ cup (125 mL) raw or cooked vegetables or 1 cup (250 mL) of raw salad greens | | |
| **4. How many servings of whole fruit do you eat per day?**<br>One serving = ½ cup (125 mL) or a medium-sized piece of whole fruit | | |
| **5. How many servings of red meat, hamburger or sausages do you eat per week?**<br>One serving = 3.5–5.5 ounces (100–150 grams) | | |
| **6. How many servings of butter, margarine or cream do you consume per day?**<br>One serving = 1 tablespoon (15 mL) | | |
| **7. How many sugar-sweetened beverages do you drink per week?**<br>One serving = 12 oz (355 mL), or one can of soda<br>Includes any drinks with added sugars (sodas, fruit drinks, sports drinks, energy drinks, iced teas, etc.) | | |
| **8. Do you drink wine? How much do you drink per week?**<br>1 glass = 5 oz (150 mL) | | |
| **9. How many servings of legumes, like kidney beans, chickpeas, lentils, black beans or split peas, do you eat per week?**<br>One serving = 5 oz (150 g), or ½–⅔ cup (125–175 mL) | | |

| MEDITERRANEAN DIET ADHERENCE SCREENER (MEDAS) | ANSWER | POINTS |
|---|---|---|
| **10. How many servings of fish or seafood do you eat per week?**<br>One serving of fish = 3.5-5.5 oz (100–156 g)<br>One serving of seafood = 7 oz (210 g) | | |
| **11. How many times do you eat baked goods such as pie, cookies, cake or doughnuts per week?** | | |
| **12. How many times do you eat nuts per week?**<br>One serving = 1 oz (30 g) | | |
| **13. Do you eat chicken or turkey more often than beef, pork, hamburger or sausage?** | | |
| **14. How many times per week do you eat dishes with a sauce of tomato, garlic and onion/leeks sautéed in olive oil?** | | |
| TOTAL POINTS: | | |

## MEDAS SCORING

**1.** Earn 1 point if your answer is yes.

**2.** Earn 1 point if your answer is ≥4 tablespoons.

**3.** Earn 1 point if your answer is ≥2 servings.

**4.** Earn 1 point if your answer is ≥3 servings.

**5.** Earn 1 point if your answer is <1 serving.

**6.** Earn 1 point if your answer is <1 serving.

**7.** Earn 1 point if your answer is <1 beverage.

**8.** Earn 1 point if your answer is ≥7 glasses.

**9.** Earn 1 point if your answer is ≥3 servings.

**10.** Earn 1 point if your answer is ≥3 servings.

**11.** Earn 1 point if your answer is <3 times.

**12.** Earn 1 point if your answer is ≥3 times.

**13.** Earn 1 point if your answer is yes.

**14.** Earn 1 point if your answer is ≥2 times.

### Score Interpretation

10–14 points out of 14 = very good adherence

6–9 points out of 14 = moderate or fair adherence

0–5 points out of 14 = weak adherence

The Mediterranean diet is considered safe for most people, and it emphasizes balance in food choices. However, some people with Parkinson's disease may need to modify the diet to accommodate swallowing difficulty and to increase caloric requirements. A change in eating habits might lead to unintentional weight loss, so adding energy-dense foods may be necessary. As with any diet, benefits may heavily depend on consistency and overall intake rather than on isolated food choices. The Mediterranean diet may be especially beneficial for individuals living with Parkinson's disease who desire a sustainable, long-term approach to supporting brain, heart and gut health.

### MEDITERRANEAN DIET CONCLUSIONS

Among the dietary patterns studied in Parkinson's disease, the Mediterranean diet has some of the strongest and most consistent evidence supporting its potential health benefits. While it is not a cure for Parkinson's disease, it provides a flexible, nutrient-rich framework that can be individualized to one's preferences and nutritional needs. It is generally a safe diet to follow as it recommends a variety of food groups and moderation.

## Mediterranean-DASH Intervention for Neurodegenerative Delay (MIND) Diet

The MIND diet is a combination of the Mediterranean diet and the Dietary Approaches to Stop Hypertension (DASH) diet. The MIND diet was originally developed to slow the decline of memory and thinking in the aging brain. The developers of the MIND diet suggest it is possibly more protective of brain health than the Mediterranean and DASH diets alone.

This diet combines specific nutrients that are associated with better brain health. Similar to the Mediterranean diet, the MIND diet emphasizes plant-based foods and limits saturated fats typically found in animal products. While it does not specifically limit salt consumption like the DASH diet, it does recommend limiting red and processed meats, similar to both the DASH and Mediterranean diets. Comparable to its foundational diets, the MIND diet also limits the addition of sugars. The MIND diet is unique in that it emphasizes green leafy vegetables and berries.

These fruits and vegetables are packed with antioxidants and polyphenols that can help to reduce oxidative stress and inflammation. Specifically:

- Nuts and seeds are high in vitamin E, a powerful antioxidant with anti-inflammatory properties.
- Dark leafy greens and whole grains are packed with B vitamins, which are essential for a healthy metabolism and proper brain cell function.
- Essential fatty acids from oily fish, like salmon and tuna, help maintain the structure of brain cells and facilitate brain-cell-to-brain-cell communication.

### MIND DIET COMPONENTS

| FOODS TO EAT | |
| --- | --- |
| Green leafy vegetables (kale, collards, greens, spinach, lettuce/tossed salad) | ≥6 servings weekly |
| Other vegetables (bell peppers, squash, carrots, broccoli, celery, potatoes, tomatoes, beets, corn, zucchini, eggplant, etc.) | ≥1 serving daily |
| Berries | ≥2 servings weekly |
| Nuts | ≥5 servings weekly |
| Cooking fat | Primarily use olive oil |
| Whole grains | ≥3 servings daily |
| Fish (not fried) | ≥1 serving weekly |
| Beans and lentils | >3 servings weekly |
| Poultry (not fried) | ≥2 servings weekly |
| **FOODS TO LIMIT** | |
| Butter or margarine | <1 tbsp (15 mL) daily |
| Cheese | <1 serving weekly |
| Red meats and processed meat products | <4 servings weekly |
| Fast fried foods | <1 time weekly |
| Pastries and sweets | <5 servings weekly |
| **ALCOHOL RECOMMENDATIONS** | |
| Wine | 1 glass daily |

Much of the research on the MIND diet has focused on cognitive decline, specifically in Alzheimer's disease and other dementias. Researchers observed people who followed the MIND diet and found that they were at a lower risk for dementia and Alzheimer's disease. This diet also slowed cognitive decline in older adults without dementia. However, whether the MIND diet has significant impacts on long-term cognition has been a hot topic of debate. In a more reliable study where researchers assigned groups to either follow the MIND diet or a control diet, there were no changes in cognition between the two groups after three years of follow-up.

When examining the small number of studies conducted on the MIND diet and Parkinson's disease risk, there appears to be a positive link between MIND diet adherence and a lower risk for later developing Parkinson's disease. However, these findings are based on observational studies, meaning we cannot conclude that the MIND diet alone lowers the risk for Parkinson's disease or changes the course of the disease itself. More research will be needed to understand how the MIND diet might impact Parkinson's disease risk and progression.

### MIND DIET CONCLUSIONS

The MIND diet is a balanced diet that contains components that support overall health. It is linked to an overall lower risk for the later development of Parkinson's disease, Alzheimer's disease and other dementias. The MIND diet is also linked to slower cognitive decline in older adults; however, its effects on long-term cognition remain unclear. The MIND diet is a sustainable diet that promotes moderation and does not eliminate entire food groups.

## Vegan and Vegetarian Diets

Vegan and vegetarian diets are plant-based diets that limit or exclude animal products. Vegetarians refrain from eating meat but may still eat products derived from animal sources, such as milk, eggs, cheese and honey. However, vegans refrain from consuming all animal-derived products, including dairy and honey. In the same vein as the MIND and Mediterranean diets, these plant-based diets have been linked to reduced inflammation and to better overall health.

Mainly studied for their effect on Parkinson's disease risk, plant-based diets are known to be high in antioxidants and in fiber. These components not only support brain health, but they also support gut health, which we have established as important for symptom management and possibly for slowing disease progression. Vegan and vegetarian diets specifically limit saturated fat, which can support cardiovascular health and further reduce the risk for comorbidities or other diseases that could complicate the Parkinson's disease process.

While research is limited, vegan and vegetarian diets fall into the plant-based diet category, which is associated with a lower risk for Parkinson's disease and possibly a slower progression of the disease. However, since most studies have been observational, we cannot conclude that the diet pattern alone is what is causing the change in risk and disease progression.

As with any diet that limits whole food groups, it is important to ensure adequate nutrient intake from other food sources. Since animal products are significant sources of vitamin $B_{12}$, people following a vegan diet may be more at risk for deficiency and may need to supplement their intake. Vegans and vegetarians must also ensure they get adequate amounts of protein from plant-based sources, such as beans, legumes, nuts, seeds and meat alternatives. Iron is less readily available from plant-based sources and so vegans and vegetarians must be careful to consume enough to meet daily requirements.

### KEY QUALITIES OF PLANT-BASED DIETS

- High in antioxidants, which helps reduce oxidative stress and inflammation
- High in fiber, which supports gut health
- Low in saturated fats, which lowers the risk for other chronic diseases

### VEGAN/ VEGETARIAN SUPPLEMENTS

- Vitamin $B_{12}$
- Vitamin D
- Iron
- Calcium
- Omega-3 fatty acids (DHA/EPA)
- Zinc
- Protein (if intake is low)

**PLANT-BASED ALTERNATIVES FOR IMPORTANT NUTRIENTS COMMONLY LACKING IN A VEGAN OR VEGETARIAN DIET**

| NUTRIENT | ANIMAL-BASED SOURCES | PLANT-BASED SOURCES |
|---|---|---|
| Vitamin $B_{12}$ | Meat, fish, poultry, eggs, dairy | Fortified foods (plant-based milks, breakfast cereals, nutritional yeast) *Vegan diets may require supplementation |
| Protein | Meat, poultry, fish, eggs, dairy | Beans, lentils, tofu, tempeh, edamame, soy milk, nuts, seeds, quinoa |
| Iron | Red meat, poultry, seafood | Lentils, beans, tofu, spinach, pumpkin seeds, fortified cereals *Pair with vitamin C to enhance absorption |
| Zinc | Meat, shellfish, dairy | Beans, lentils, whole grains, seeds |
| Calcium | Milk, yogurt, cheese | Fortified plant-based milks, calcium-set tofu, tahini, almonds, leafy greens |
| Vitamin D | Fatty fish, egg yolks, fortified dairy | Fortified plant-based milks, UV-exposed mushrooms *Diet may require supplementation |

## FAQ: SHOULD I AVOID MILK?

While dairy is a great source of important nutrients, dairy consumption is an ongoing debate in the world of Parkinson's disease. In observational studies, higher consumption of low-fat dairy products has been linked to an increased risk for developing Parkinson's. This association is mainly linked to low-fat and non-fat milk intake rather than consumption of fermented dairy products, like yogurt and cheese. While not fully understood, some researchers suggest dairy may lower uric acid levels, resulting in lower levels of antioxidants. Other researchers suggest dairy could be a vehicle for increased pesticide or other toxic compound exposure. Either way, the research is very limited and primarily based on observation. Again, this means we cannot draw strong conclusions about whether dairy intake does more harm than good.

It is likely most beneficial to consume dairy in moderation. It remains an important source of nutrients, like vitamin D and calcium, that are important for bone health and overall well-being.

## THE BETTER CHOICE: ORGANIC VERSUS CONVENTIONAL

Given the link between environmental exposures, like pesticides, and the increased risk of Parkinson's disease, the debate of whether one should choose organic versus conventional foods is highly relevant.

**What is organic?**

Organic foods are tightly regulated by standards that include using eco-friendly pest control and natural fertilizers when growing produce, raising livestock without the use of antibiotics and growth hormones, and ensuring packaged goods are free of artificial colors and preservatives. People choose organic foods for a variety of reasons, including food safety, health, environmental concerns, animal welfare and differences in taste and quality. However, barriers remain to purchasing organic, as these foods often are more costly and have limited availability.

**What does the research say?**

Whether or not organic is "healthier" than conventional remains poorly understood. Some studies show health benefits from eating organic produce. However, when examining studies that compare organic versus conventional, it is hard to determine if health benefits are due to eating organic produce or because of a combination of factors resulting from the consumer's lifestyle. For example, people that choose organic may be more health-conscious and as a result follow a healthier diet and make healthier choices in the other areas of life, such as going to preventive wellness visits and following physical activity recommendations. While some studies show benefits from choosing organic, others show no difference in health outcomes.

**What is the bottom line?**

There is not enough solid evidence to recommend one over the other. If your budget allows for choosing organic and you have access to it, great! If your circumstances point you toward conventional, that's also fine! No matter the source of your produce, you should always wash it thoroughly before eating to remove dirt, bacteria and pesticide residue.

**How to wash produce:**

1. Wash your hands for at least 20 seconds with soap and warm water.
2. Rinse produce before you peel it. This prevents residue on the outside of the produce from being transferred to other areas.
3. Gently rub produce under running water. For tougher foods, like melons, use a vegetable brush to scrub under running water.
4. Dry produce with a clean cloth. Remove the outermost leaves of leafy produce, like a head of lettuce.

## References

Academy of Nutrition and Dietetics. Celiac Disease (2023): Nutrition Intervention. Nutrition Care Manual. Updated 2023. Accessed November 15, 2025. https://www.nutritioncaremanual.org/topic.cfm?ncm_category_id=1&lv1=5522&lv2=275278&lv3=275289&ncm_toc_id=275289&ncm_heading=Nutrition%20Care.

Ansari U, Omid A, Nadora D, et al. Outcomes of dietary interventions in the prevention and progression of Parkinson's disease: A literature review. *AIMS Neurosci.* 2024 Dec 30;11(4):520-532. doi: 10.3934/Neuroscience.2024032. PMID: 39801794; PMCID: PMC11712231.

Anwar L, Ahmad E, Imtiaz M, et al. The Impact of Diet on Parkinson's Disease: A Systematic Review. Cureus. 2024 Sep 27;16(9):e70337. doi: 10.7759/cureus.70337. PMID: 39469346; PMCID: PMC11513219.

Barnes LL, Dhana K, Liu X, et al. Trial of the MIND Diet for Prevention of Cognitive Decline in Older Persons. *N Engl J Med.* 2023 Aug 17;389(7):602-611. doi: 10.1056/NEJMoa2302368. Epub 2023 Jul 18. PMID: 37466280; PMCID: PMC10513737.

Bohnen JLB, Albin RL, Bohnen NI. Ketogenic interventions in mild cognitive impairment, Alzheimer's disease, and Parkinson's disease: A systematic review and critical appraisal. *Front Neurol.* 2023 Feb 9;14:1123290. doi: 10.3389/fneur.2023.1123290. PMID: 36846143; PMCID: PMC9947355.

Gantenbein KV, Kanaka-Gantenbein C. Mediterranean Diet as an Antioxidant: The Impact on Metabolic Health and Overall Wellbeing. *Nutrients.* 2021 Jun 6;13(6):1951. doi: 10.3390/nu13061951. PMID: 34204057; PMCID: PMC8227318.

Hamilton Health Sciences. Mediterranean Diet Adherence Screener (MEDAS). 2022. Accessed 2025 September 22. https://www.hamiltonhealthsciences.ca/wp-content/uploads/2022/04/Cardiac-Health-Mediterranean-Diet-Adherence-Screener.pdf.

Harvard T.H. Chan School of Public Health. Diet Review: Ketogenic Diet for Weight Loss. The Nutrition Source. 2026. Accessed January 15, 2026. https://nutritionsource.hsph.harvard.edu/healthy-weight/diet-reviews/ketogenic-diet/.

Klann EM, Dissanayake U, Gurrala A, et al. The Gut-Brain Axis and Its Relation to Parkinson's Disease: A Review. *Front Aging Neurosci.* 2022 Jan 7;13:782082. doi: 10.3389/fnagi.2021.782082. PMID: 35069178; PMCID: PMC8776990.

Komati N, Cravedi JP, Lecerf JM, et al. Potential Health Benefits of a Diet Rich in Organic Fruit and Vegetables versus a Diet Based on Conventional Produce: A Systematic Review. *Nutr Rev.* 2025 Mar 1;83(3):e1101-e1114. doi: 10.1093/nutrit/nuae104. PMID: 39101594; PMCID: PMC11819487.

Morris MC, Tangney CC, Wang Y, et al. MIND diet slows cognitive decline with aging. *Alzheimers Dement.* 2015 Sep;11(9):1015-22. doi: 10.1016/j.jalz.2015.04.011. Epub 2015 Jun 15. PMID: 26086182; PMCID: PMC4581900.

Muttalib Z, Aboukhalil D, Nwosu C, et al. Gluten and its relationship with inflammation and Parkinson's Disease: A literature review. *AIMS Neurosci.* 2025 Mar 31;12(1):44-57. doi: 10.3934/Neuroscience.2025004. PMID: 40270951; PMCID: PMC12011982.

Rusch C, Beke M, Nieves C Jr, et al. Promotion of a Mediterranean Diet Alters Constipation Symptoms and Fecal Calprotectin in People with Parkinson's Disease: A Randomized Controlled Trial. *Nutrients.* 2024 Sep 2;16(17):2946. doi: 10.3390/nu16172946. PMID: 39275262; PMCID: PMC11396875.

Seelarbokus BA, Menozzi E, Schapira AHV, et al. Mediterranean Diet Adherence, Gut Microbiota and Parkinson's Disease: A Systematic Review. *Nutrients*. 2024 Jul 9;16(14):2181. doi: 10.3390/nu16142181. PMID: 39064625; PMCID: PMC11280252.

Solch RJ, Aigbogun JO, Voyiadjis AG, et al. Mediterranean diet adherence, gut microbiota, and Alzheimer's or Parkinson's disease risk: A systematic review. *J Neurol Sci*. 2022 Mar 15;434:120166. doi: 10.1016/j.jns.2022.120166. Epub 2022 Jan 26. PMID: 35144237.

Tosefsky KN, Zhu J, Wang YN, et al. The Role of Diet in Parkinson's Disease. *J Parkinsons Dis*. 2024;14(s1):S21-S34. doi: 10.3233/JPD-230264. PMID: 38251061; PMCID: PMC11380239.

U.S. Department of Agriculture. USDA Certified Organic: Understanding the Basics. Agriculture Marketing Service. 2026. Accessed January 17, 2026. https://www.ams.usda.gov/services/organic-certification/organic-basics.

U.S. Food and Drug Administration. 7 Tips for Cleaning Fruits, Vegetables. Updated June 15, 2021. Accessed January 17, 2026. https://www.fda.gov/consumers/consumerupdates/7-tips-cleaning-fruits-vegetables.

van Soest AP, Beers S, van de Rest O, et al. The Mediterranean-Dietary Approaches to Stop Hypertension Intervention for Neurodegenerative Delay (MIND) Diet for the Aging Brain: A Systematic Review. Adv Nutr. 2024 Mar;15(3):100184. doi: 10.1016/j.advnut.2024.100184. Epub 2024 Feb 3. PMID: 38311314; PMCID: PMC10942868.

CHAPTER 8

# DIETARY SUPPLEMENTS

*Supplements are meant to be added to the diet rather than to replace a balanced diet.*

Dietary supplements are products containing vitamins, minerals, herbs, botanicals or other combinations of products. Supplements are meant to be added to the diet rather than to replace a balanced diet. Typically, dietary supplements are heavily advertised for their health benefits; however, they are not intended to treat or to cure diseases. Not all dietary supplements on the market have proven benefits that outweigh risks. Supplements are not regulated the same way medications are, and supplements have the potential to interact with medications one might already be taking. Taking certain supplements at high doses can result in adverse effects. This chapter reviews the benefits and risks of some, but not all, supplements studied for their effectiveness in Parkinson's disease.

## HOMOCYSTEINE LEVELS

Taking levodopa can lead to higher levels of homocysteine in the body. Homocysteine is a type of amino acid important for the role it plays in metabolism, but too much homocysteine has been linked to osteoporosis, cognitive decline, cardiovascular problems and oxidative stress. Certain B vitamins play an important role in reducing homocysteine levels.

## Vitamins

| VITAMIN | RECOMMENDED AMOUNTS |
| --- | --- |
| Vitamin A | 700-900mcg/day (adults >18 years) |
| Vitamin $B_6$ | 1.3mg/day (adults 19-50 years)<br>1.7mg/day (men >51 years)<br>1.5mg/day (women >51 years) |
| Vitamin $B_9$ (Folate) | 400mcg DFEs/day (dietary folate equivalents) (adults >18 years) |
| Vitamin $B_{12}$ | 2.4mcg/day (adults >18 years) |
| Vitamin C | 75mg/day (women >18 years)<br>90mg/day (men >18 years) |
| Vitamin D | 15mcg/day (adults 19-70 years)<br>20mcg/day (>70 years) |
| Vitamin E | 15mg/day (adults >18 years) |

### Vitamin $B_6$

Vitamin $B_6$ plays an important role in reducing homocysteine levels. Adults aged 19 to 50 years should aim for 1.3 mg/day. Men over 51 years of age should aim for 1.7 mg/day, and women over 51 years of age should aim for 1.5 mg/day. Vitamin $B_6$ can be found in foods like fish, chickpeas, beef liver, potatoes and fortified cereals. Vitamin $B_6$ deficiency is not common as most people consume enough from their diet and/or a multivitamin.

High-dose supplementation is not generally recommended. High doses of vitamin $B_6$ have been linked to poor medication effectiveness especially if levodopa is taken without carbidopa. Many patients taking a combination of levodopa and carbidopa will maintain reasonable vitamin $B_6$ levels. High doses of vitamin $B_6$ should be avoided as they can lead to nerve damage and numb feet. Your primary care doctor should monitor your vitamin $B_6$ level each year if you have Parkinson's.

### Vitamin $B_9$ (Folate)

Folate plays an important role in reducing homocysteine levels. Most adults should aim for 400 mcg of dietary folate equivalents (DFEs) per day from food sources like dark leafy green vegetables, fruits, dairy, poultry, nuts and beans. Cereals and grains typically have added folate to prevent deficiencies in the American population. Most adults consume enough folate from the diet; however, a multivitamin containing folate can also help to meet the recommended intake if deficiency is identified. Too much folate can mask vitamin $B_{12}$ deficiency.

### Vitamin $B_{12}$

Vitamin $B_{12}$ plays an important role in reducing homocysteine levels. Older adults are at an elevated risk for vitamin $B_{12}$ deficiency, which has been associated with cognitive decline and faster progression of symptoms in those living with Parkinson's disease. Most adults should aim for 2.4 mcg per day from food sources like meats, poultry, fish, eggs and dairy products. Additional supplementation is recommended if you are on dopamine replacement therapy. In this case, a multivitamin or B-complex vitamin may be recommended. For adults that have problems absorbing vitamin $B_{12}$, a $B_{12}$ injection may be necessary. Having your doctor check a $B_{12}$ level every year is important if you have Parkinson's.

### Vitamin C

Vitamin C is an antioxidant important for getting rid of free radicals and supporting the immune system. Given the link between oxidative stress and Parkinson's disease, antioxidants like vitamin C have been studied for how they might impact brain health. While some studies show a link between consuming enough vitamin C and a lower risk of developing Parkinson's disease, whether supplementing with vitamin C following the diagnosis of Parkinson's disease changes the outcome remains poorly investigated. Most people consume enough vitamin C from fruits and vegetables and do not require supplementation.

### Vitamin D

Adequate vitamin D intake is important for muscle function and bone health. It has also been associated with improved mood and cognition in older adults. Research shows people living with Parkinson's disease are more likely to have low levels of vitamin D, possibly due to decreased sun exposure, aging and inadequate intake. Lower levels of vitamin D are associated with worse balance and an increased risk of falls and fractures. Whether or not low vitamin D levels cause these issues or if they are simply correlated with the lifestyle leading to these issues is unknown. For example, someone that has limited mobility might restrict outdoor activities, leading to less sun exposure and lower vitamin D levels but also leading to limited physical activity that could increase the risk for fractures. Most experts believe that vitamin D deficiency in the setting of Parkinson's is an actual biological part of the illness.

Adults generally need 15 mcg of vitamin D per day, and this number increases to 20 mcg per day after the age of 70. Vitamin D is found naturally in fatty fish, cod liver oil, beef liver, egg yolks and mushrooms. Fortified foods also provide vitamin D, and these foods include milk and milk alternatives, cheese, ice cream, yogurt, breakfast cereals and orange juice.

There is limited research on vitamin D supplementation for those living with Parkinson's disease. Without strong evidence that vitamin D could alter the course of the disease, regular supplementation is not generally recommended. For people who are deficient in vitamin D or are at an increased risk for osteoporosis and falls, vitamin D supplementation may be recommended.

### Vitamin E

Vitamin E is a type of antioxidant that protects cells from oxidative stress. Since oxidative stress is a component of Parkinson's disease, vitamin E has been studied for how it might impact the progression of the disease. While higher intakes of vitamin E have been associated with a lower risk for developing Parkinson's disease, large-scale studies show no association between vitamin E supplementation and improvements in symptoms or disease progression. Therefore, vitamin E supplementation is not generally required. Adequate vitamin E intake is encouraged from food sources like nuts, seeds, avocados and vegetable oils. High-dose vitamin E supplementation can interfere with blood thinners and may increase bleeding risk.

## Minerals

| MINERAL | RECOMMENDED AMOUNTS |
|---|---|
| Calcium | 1,000mg/day (men 19-70 years; women 19-50 years)<br>1,200mg/day (men >70 years; women >50 years) |
| Iron | 8mg/day (men >18 years; women >50 years)<br>18mg/day (women 19-50 years) |
| Zinc | 8-11mg/day (adults >18 years) |
| Potassium | ~2,600-3,400mg (adults >18 years) |

### Calcium

Calcium is an essential mineral important for bone health, muscle function, and nerve communication. For people living with Parkinson's disease, calcium is especially important for its role in maintaining bone density and preventing fractures from falls. While not generally recommended in supplemental form, a supplement may be helpful for those that are unable to consume enough calcium through their diet or that are at a greater risk for osteoporosis. Both men and women are at greater risk for osteoporosis with Parkinson's. Men should aim for 1,000 mg/day, and this number increases to 1,200 mg/day after the age of 70. Women should aim for 1,000 mg/day, and this number increases to 1,200 mg/day after the age of 50. Adults should be careful not to consume more than 2,000 to 2,500 mg of calcium per day as this can increase the risk for developing kidney stones. Calcium supplements can interact with some medications, such as levothyroxine, lithium and certain antibiotics.

#### KEY FOOD SOURCES OF CALCIUM

Dairy products, like milk, cheese and yogurt, are great sources of calcium. Some milk substitutes, like soymilk, have added calcium. Other food sources include canned fish with bones, kale and broccoli.

### Iron

Iron is a trace mineral important for helping transport oxygen to vital organs. Too little iron can lead to health consequences; however, higher intakes of dietary iron have been associated with an increased risk for Parkinson's disease. Excessive levels of iron in the brain can lead to oxidative stress and damage to dopaminergic neurons, the brain cells that are damaged in Parkinson's disease. People living with the disease should aim for a healthy balance of dietary iron as they may be at risk for deficiency.

Men aged 19 years or older and women aged 51 years or older should aim for 8 mg/day of iron. Women aged 19 to

50 years old should aim for 18 mg/day. People that do not eat meat require more as iron from plant sources is not as readily absorbed compared to iron from animal sources. Adults should not exceed 45 mg/day of iron from food and supplements.

While routine iron supplementation is not generally recommended for people living with Parkinson's disease, your health-care team may recommend supplementation if you have iron deficiency. Iron deficiency is more common in older adults, especially those with gastrointestinal problems like constipation and gastroparesis.

Iron supplements can interfere with levodopa absorption especially if taken at the same time. If your health-care team has recommended an iron supplement, it is best to space the supplement and levodopa at least 2 hours apart.

**KEY FOOD SOURCES OF IRON**

Meats, including beef, lamb and liver; legumes, including lentils, beans and chickpeas; whole grains; and leafy greens including spinach and Swiss chard.

## Antioxidants & Neuroprotective Compounds

### Alpha-Lipoic Acid

Alpha-lipoic acid (ALA) is an antioxidant that helps with mitochondrial functioning. It has been studied in other neurological disorders, including Alzheimer's disease, and it may have some benefit on cognitive decline. However, studies on the neuroprotective effects of ALA in Parkinson's disease have been limited to animal models. Currently, there is not enough evidence to recommend supplementation for humans.

**KEY FOOD SOURCES OF ANTIOXIDANTS**

Spinach, broccoli, Brussels sprouts, tomatoes, carrots, potatoes, avocado, berries, beets, soy products, lean meats, fatty fish, olive oil, nuts, garlic . . . to name a few!

### Coenzyme Q10

Coenzyme Q10 (CoQ10) acts as an antioxidant and plays a role in cellular energy production. CoQ10 is found naturally in meat, fish, nuts and some oils. Recent findings suggest that people living with Parkinson's disease could have lower levels of CoQ10 in the body. Early studies examining CoQ10 supplementation in Parkinson's disease were promising; however, more recent large-scale studies have not revealed a benefit of CoQ10 supplements on disease progression or motor symptoms. While not recommended to treat Parkinson's disease, CoQ10 supplementation is generally considered safe. Higher doses may cause insomnia or gastrointestinal upset.

## ESSENTIAL FATTY ACIDS

**Omega-3 fatty acids (EPA/DHA)**

Omega-3 fatty acids are types of polyunsaturated fatty acids that are essential in the diet. Much of the research on omega-3s centers on three types: alphalipoic acid (ALA), eicosapentaenoic acid (EPA) and docosahexaenoic acid (DHA). These fatty acids play a role in reducing inflammation and supporting communication between brain cells. While research has been limited to a very small number of studies, preliminary evidence suggests a beneficial effect against Parkinson's progression when omega-3 supplementation is given congruently with vitamin E. This was demonstrated by better Parkinson's symptom scores, less oxidative stress, better mood and reduced inflammatory markers. While promising, more research is needed before regular supplementation is recommended.

Omega-3 fatty acids can be found in fatty fish, like salmon, tuna and sardines, and fish oils. They can also be found in plant oils, like flaxseed, soybean and canola oils. Supplemental forms are also available and are relatively safe. Higher doses (>900 mg/day of EPA plus 600 mg/day DHA or more for several weeks) should be avoided as they have the potential to suppress the immune system. Supplemental forms may also increase the risk of bleeding, especially when taken with warfarin, or Coumadin.

### Glutathione

Glutathione is a type of antioxidant that gained interest as a potential therapy after evidence revealed reduced levels of glutathione in the brains of those with Parkinson's disease. Glutathione has been important for reducing oxidative stress and supporting energy production in cells. Researchers theorized that since glutathione levels were lower in Parkinson's disease, supplementation might help to protect brain cells from damage. However, to date there are no substantial studies revealing significant changes in the disease process or progression that result from glutathione supplementation.

## Herbs & Botanical Extracts

Various herbs and botanicals have been studied for their effectiveness in Parkinson's disease. However, there is currently not enough evidence to suggest their regular usage. Many of these products are accompanied by adverse effects and may interfere with certain medications, including blood thinners.

### Curcumin (turmeric)

Curcumin is a component of turmeric, a plant in the ginger family. In animal studies, curcumin has been shown to reduce oxidative stress, inflammation and the accumulation of $\alpha$-synuclein, the protein that is misfolded in Parkinson's disease. Curcumin was also linked to a slower progression of motor symptoms. While these animal studies show promising results, we cannot conclude that the same would be true in humans. Since there is not enough research looking at curcumin supplementation in people living with Parkinson's disease, it is not currently recommended as a treatment.

While not studied for safety, particularly in those living with Parkinson's disease, conventional curcumin supplements are likely safe for up to 2 to 3 months. However, formulations marketed for their increased bioavailability have the potential to cause liver damage. Additionally, oral turmeric may lead to gastrointestinal upset.

## Probiotics & Digestive Health

Probiotics are live microorganisms, mainly bacteria, that provide health benefits for the host. Since there has been an observed shift in the gut microbiome of people living with Parkinson's disease, research focusing on ways to correct this imbalance has included the use of probiotics. Probiotics are available in fermented food products, like yogurt and kefir, and also in supplements. Certain foods, like milk, nutrition bars and smoothies, can be formulated with added probiotics. These additions are usually marked on the label. Supplements are available in a wide variety of strains and potencies and are usually in pill, liquid or powder form.

Probiotics have been shown to be beneficial in a subset of healthy adults with functional constipation. However, studies looking specifically at probiotic use in adults with Parkinson's disease have been limited. Most of the research focuses on probiotics and their effect on constipation rather than their effect on Parkinson's disease itself. Researchers have suggested that strains of *Lactobacillus*, *Akkermansia* and *Bifidobacterium* may be most beneficial. While likely safe, research on probiotic use in Parkinson's disease has not been concrete enough to encourage regular use. The side effects of probiotic use may include gassiness and bloating.

### FOOD SOURCES OF PROBIOTICS

- Some cheeses
- Yogurt
- Kefir
- Kimchi
- Kombucha
- Sauerkraut
- Miso
- Pickles
- Raw unfiltered apple cider vinegar
- Foods with probiotics added during processing (indicated on food label)

## Metabolic and Cellular Support

### Creatine

It is known that creatine supplementation combined with exercise can improve muscle performance and strength. There is some evidence that creatine supplementation could improve thinking and cognition outside of Parkinson's disease. However, long-term studies in people living with Parkinson's disease have failed to reveal that creatine has an appreciable effect on disease progression.

### UNDERSTANDING CREATINE

Creatine is a naturally occurring compound found in muscle and brain cells that helps produce energy. It plays a role in supporting cellular energy systems and has been studied for potential benefits in muscle function and neurological health, though its role in Parkinson's remains under investigation.

### Nicotinamide Riboside/NAD+ Precursors

Nicotinamide adenine dinucleotide (NAD) is an important molecule in mitochondrial function. NAD supplementation in animal models has revealed protective effects against neurodegeneration. The NADPARK study showed that an NAD precursor, nicotinamide riboside (NR), increased brain NAD levels with supplementation of 1,000 mg for 30 days. This increase was associated with clinical improvement in a subgroup of participants. More studies are needed to confirm these findings and the safety of NR supplementation before it can be recommended.

## References


Agnieszka W, Paweł P, Małgorzata K. How to Optimize the Effectiveness and Safety of Parkinson's Disease Therapy? - A Systematic Review of Drugs Interactions with Food and Dietary Supplements. *Curr Neuropharmacol.* 2022;20(7):1427-1447. doi: 10.2174/1570159X19666211116142806. PMID: 34784871; PMCID: PMC9881082.

Boelens Keun JT, Arnoldussen IA, Vriend C, et al. Dietary Approaches to Improve Efficacy and Control Side Effects of Levodopa Therapy in Parkinson's Disease: A Systematic Review. *Adv Nutr.* 2021 Dec 1;12(6):2265-2287. doi: 10.1093/advances/nmab060. PMID: 34113965; PMCID: PMC8634393.

Brakedal B, Dölle C, Riemer F, et al. The NADPARK study: A randomized phase I trial of nicotinamide riboside supplementation in Parkinson's disease. *Cell Metab.* 2022 Mar 1;34(3):396-407.e6. doi: 10.1016/j.cmet.2022.02.001. PMID: 35235774.

Chang YH. Curcumin as a potential therapeutic agent for Parkinson's disease: a systematic review. *Front Pharmacol.* 2025 Apr 22;16:1593191. doi: 10.3389/fphar.2025.1593191. PMID: 40331193; PMCID: PMC12052530.

Detopoulou P, Voulgaridou G, Saridaki A, et al. Omega-3 fatty acids' supplementation in Parkinson's disease: A systematic review of randomized controlled trials. *Clin Nutr Open Sci.* 2024 Jun;55:P102-115. doi: 10.1016/j.nutos.2024.03.007.

Ghalandari N, Assarzadegan F, Mahdavi H, et al. Evaluating the effectiveness of probiotics in relieving constipation in Parkinson's disease: A systematic review and meta-analysis. *Heliyon.* 2023 Mar 4;9(3):e14312. doi: 10.1016/j.heliyon.2023.e14312. PMID: 36938477; PMCID: PMC10015253.

Gutiérrez-Hellín J, Del Coso J, Franco-Andrés A, et al. Creatine Supplementation Beyond Athletics: Benefits of Different Types of Creatine for Women, Vegans, and Clinical Populations-A Narrative Review. *Nutrients.* 2024 Dec 29;17(1):95. doi: 10.3390/nu17010095. PMID: 39796530; PMCID: PMC11723027.

Homann CN, Homann B, Ivanic G, Urbanic-Purkart T. Vitamin D supplementation in later life: a systematic review of efficacy and safety in movement disorders. *Front Aging Neurosci.* 2024 Jan 26;16:1333217. doi: 10.3389/fnagi.2024.1333217. PMID: 38343878; PMCID: PMC10853433.

Liu L, Shen Q, Bao Y, et al. Association between dietary intake and risk of Parkinson's disease: cross-sectional analysis of survey data from NHANES 2007-2016. *Front Nutr.* 2023 Dec 15;10:1278128. doi: 10.3389/fnut.2023.1278128. PMID: 38192644; PMCID: PMC10773772.

Mantle D, Hargreaves IP. Mitochondrial Dysfunction and Neurodegenerative Disorders: Role of Nutritional Supplementation. *Int J Mol Sci.* 2022 Oct 20;23(20):12603. doi: 10.3390/ijms232012603. PMID: 36293457; PMCID: PMC9604531.

Niu C, Dong M, Niu Y. Role of Glutathione in Parkinson's Disease Pathophysiology and Therapeutic Potential of Polyphenols. *Phytother Res.* 2024 Dec;38(12):5567-5582. doi: 10.1002/ptr.8342. Epub 2024 Sep 17. PMID: 39290049.

Rauchová H. Coenzyme Q10 effects in neurological diseases. *Physiol Res.* 2021 Dec 30;70(Suppl4):S683-S714. doi: 10.33549/physiolres.934712. PMID: 35199552; PMCID: PMC9054193.

U.S. Department of Health and Human Services. Calcium Fact Sheet for Health Professionals. National Institutes of Health Office of Dietary Supplements. Updated July 11, 2025. Accessed January 15, 2026. https://ods.od.nih.gov/factsheets/calcium-HealthProfessional/.

U.S. Department of Health and Human Services. Coenzyme Q10. National Center for Complementary and Integrative Health. Updated January 2019. Accessed January 13, 2026. https://www.nccih.nih.gov/health/coenzyme-q10.

U.S. Department of Health and Human Services. Dietary Supplements: What You Need to Know. National Institutes of Health Office of Dietary Supplements. Updated January 4, 2023. Accessed January 6, 2026. https://ods.od.nih.gov/factsheets/WYNTK-Consumer/.

U.S. Department of Health and Human Services. Folate Fact Sheet for Health Professionals. National Institutes of Health Office of Dietary Supplements. Updated November 30, 2022. Accessed January 30, 2026. https://ods.od.nih.gov/factsheets/Folate-HealthProfessional/.

U.S. Department of Health and Human Services. Iron Fact Sheet for Health Professionals. National Institutes of Health Office of Dietary Supplements. Updated September 4, 2025. Accessed January 14, 2026. https://ods.od.nih.gov/factsheets/Iron-HealthProfessional/#h9.

U.S. Department of Health and Human Services. Omega-3 Fatty Acids Fact Sheet for Health Professionals. National Institutes of Health Office of Dietary Supplements. Updated August 22, 2025. Accessed January 20, 2026. https://ods.od.nih.gov/factsheets/Omega3FattyAcids-HealthProfessional/.

U.S. Department of Health and Human Services. Probiotics Fact Sheet for Health Professionals. National Institutes of Health Office of Dietary Supplements. Updated March 25, 2025. Accessed January 21, 2026. https://ods.od.nih.gov/factsheets/Probiotics-HealthProfessional/.

U.S. Department of Health and Human Services. Turmeric. National Center for Complementary and Integrative Health. Updated April 2025. Accessed January 14, 2026. https://www.nccih.nih.gov/health/turmeric.

U.S. Department of Health and Human Services. Vitamin $B_{12}$ Fact Sheet for Health Professionals. National Institutes of Health Office of Dietary Supplements. Updated July 2, 2025. Accessed January 30, 2026. https://ods.od.nih.gov/factsheets/VitaminB12-HealthProfessional/.

U.S. Department of Health and Human Services. Vitamin $B_6$ Fact Sheet for Health Professionals. National Institutes of Health Office of Dietary Supplements. Updated June 16, 2023. Accessed January 30, 2026. https://ods.od.nih.gov/factsheets/VitaminB6-HealthProfessional/#h18.

U.S. Department of Health and Human Services. Vitamin D Fact Sheet for Health Professionals. National Institutes of Health Office of Dietary Supplements. Updated June 27, 2025. Accessed January 14, 2026. https://ods.od.nih.gov/factsheets/VitaminD-HealthProfessional/.

U.S. Department of Health and Human Services. Vitamin E Fact Sheet for Health Professionals. National Institutes of Health Office of Dietary Supplements. Updated March 26, 2021. Accessed January 14, 2026. https://ods.od.nih.gov/factsheets/VitaminE-HealthProfessional/.

PART IV

# RECIPES FOR PEOPLE LIVING WITH PARKINSON'S DISEASE

CHAPTER 9

# MEAL PLANNING AND PREPARATION

*This chapter focuses on practical strategies to transform meal planning and preparation into a safer and more manageable set of tasks.*

Parkinson's symptoms can make meal planning, grocery shopping and meal preparation difficult. Tasks such as chopping foods, lifting cookware and standing for longer periods of time are frequently complicated by tremor and rigidity. Non-motor symptoms, such as fatigue, forgetfulness and fluctuations in appetite can further complicate your decisions about what and when to eat. This chapter focuses on practical strategies to transform meal planning and preparation into a safer and more manageable set of tasks.

## Step 1: Meal Planning

The first step in preparing meals is to plan ahead. Keep meals simple and predictable by rotating a small set of familiar recipes. This method can help to reduce decision-making fatigue. It may be helpful to plan "mix-and-match" meals that can be easily modified. For example, stock components like grains, proteins and vegetables that can be rotated, rather than getting caught up in planning an elaborate recipe. Alternatively, you could plan to bulk-cook by making larger quantities to freeze for later. This saves time and effort during the daily meal preparation process.

### MIX-AND-MATCH MEAL EXAMPLES

| PROTEIN | GRAIN | VEGETABLE |
|---|---|---|
| Beans, peas, lentils | Brown or wild rice | Leafy greens |
| Tofu, tempeh | Quinoa | Carrots |
| Chicken, turkey | Whole wheat pasta | Broccoli |
| Fresh or canned fish | Farro, barley, risotto | Cauliflower |
| Red meat (limit) | Flatbread, tortilla | Sweet potato |
| Eggs, dairy | Whole-grain toast | Onion and bell peppers |

## Step 2: Grocery Shopping

Once you have a plan in place, it's time to start implementing that plan. These days, there are many ways to grocery shop that can help save time and money. For those with limited time and energy or for those that have difficulty with transportation to the grocery store, ordering groceries online and utilizing delivery services or curbside pickup may be the most efficient option. Be sure to have a grocery list that you have created focused on the meals you have planned, whether you're shopping in-person or online. If shopping in-person, organize your list by the sections in the grocery store to avoid having to go back and forth. Many grocery stores provide recipe resources that you can use to help your grocery shopping and to assist you with developing an overall meal plan goal.

## Step 3: Meal Preparation

Once you have your kitchen and pantry stocked, it's time to get cooking. To save energy, use convenient foods strategically. Pre-cut produce, frozen vegetables, low-sodium canned beans and rotisserie chicken are all great examples of convenience foods that can be used to create healthy meals. Store commonly used ingredients at eye levels and within easy reach to reduce bending, lifting and searching. Use adaptive kitchen equipment when needed. Energy-saving equipment might include a slow cooker, pressure cooker, food processor, air fryer, electric can opener and an adaptive jar opener. Equipment that can help improve safety might include nonslip mats, weighted or built-up utensils, a food chopper or adaptive cutting tools. Be sure to involve friends and family to help to make the meal preparation process less burdensome and more enjoyable.

## Step 4: Focus on Food Safety

Older adults are at a higher risk for foodborne illness, so it is important to follow safe food practices when preparing, cooking and storing food. Four simple steps can help ensure food safety:

### 1. Clean: Wash Hands, Utensils and Surfaces Often

Before, during and after handling food, wash your hands with soap and water for 20 seconds. Be sure to rinse thoroughly and to dry your hands with a clean towel. Wash fruits and vegetables before use, and use a produce brush to scrub firm produce, like melons. Fruits and vegetables commonly have pesticides from the fields remaining on their surface. Make sure to wash copiously or use a vegetable wash. Don't wash raw meat, poultry or seafood as this practice can spread germs to other kitchen surfaces.

### 2. Separate: Don't Cross-Contaminate

Use a separate cutting board for raw meat, poultry and seafood. Ready-to-eat raw fruits and vegetables should be prepared using a separate cutting board. Use separate plates and utensils for raw and cooked foods.

### 3. Cook to the Right Temperature

Using a food thermometer, test the temperature of the thickest part of the food product to be sure the food is safe to eat before serving. See the proper cooking temperatures chart below.

| PRODUCT | MINIMUM INTERNAL TEMPERATURE |
|---|---|
| All poultry, including ground<br>Reheating fully cooked ham<br>Leftovers<br>Casseroles | 165°F (74°C) |
| Ground meats<br>Eggs | 160°F (71°C) |
| Beef, pork, veal and lamb (steaks, chops and roasts)<br>Ham, fresh or smoked (uncooked) | 145°F (63°C) and let rest for at least 3 minutes |
| Fish and shellfish | 145°F (63°C) |

### 4. Chill: Refrigerate and Freeze Food Properly

Place leftovers in shallow containers and refrigerate them promptly. Perishable foods should not be left out of the refrigerator for longer than 2 hours. See the chart on the next page for safe storage times and temperatures for various foods.

| FOOD | TYPE | REFRIGERATOR (40°F/4°C OR BELOW) | FREEZER (0°F/−18°C OR BELOW) |
|---|---|---|---|
| Prepared Salads | Egg, chicken, ham, tuna and macaroni salads | 3 to 4 days | Does not freeze well |
| Hot dogs | Opened package | 1 week | 1 to 2 months |
| | Unopened package | 2 weeks | 1 to 2 months |
| Luncheon meat | Opened package or deli sliced | 3 to 5 days | 1 to 2 months |
| | Unopened package | 2 weeks | 1 to 2 months |
| Bacon and sausage | Bacon | 1 week | 1 month |
| | Sausage, raw, from chicken, turkey, pork or beef | 1 to 2 days | 1 to 2 months |
| | Sausage, fully cooked, from chicken, turkey, pork or beef | 1 week | 1 to 2 months |
| | Sausage, purchased frozen | After cooking, 3 to 4 days | 1 to 2 months from date of purchase |
| Hamburger, ground meats and ground poultry | Hamburger, ground beef, turkey, chicken, other poultry, veal, pork, lamb and mixtures of these | 1 to 2 days | 3 to 4 months |
| Fresh beef, veal, lamb and pork | Steaks | 3 to 5 days | 4 to 12 months |
| | Chops | 3 to 5 days | 4 to 12 months |
| | Roasts | 3 to 5 days | 4 to 12 months |
| Ham | Fresh, uncured, uncooked | 3 to 5 days | 6 months |
| | Fresh, uncured, cooked | 3 to 4 days | 3 to 4 months |
| | Cured, cook-before-eating, uncooked | 5 to 7 days or "use by" date | 3 to 4 months |

| FOOD | TYPE | REFRIGERATOR (40°F/4°C OR BELOW) | FREEZER (0°F/−18°C OR BELOW) |
|---|---|---|---|
| Ham *(continued)* | Fully cooked, vacuum-sealed at plant, unopened | 2 weeks or "use by" date | 1 to 2 months |
| | Cooked, store-wrapped, whole | 1 week | 1 to 2 months |
| | Cooked, store-wrapped, slices, half or spiral cut | 3 to 5 days | 1 to 2 months |
| | Country ham, cooked | 1 week | 1 month |
| | Canned, labeled "keep refrigerated," unopened | 6 to 9 months | Do not freeze |
| | Canned, shelf-stable, opened<br>Note: an unopened, shelf-stable canned ham can be stored at room temperature for 2 years. | 3 to 4 days | 1 to 2 months |
| | Prosciutto, parma or serrano ham, dry Italian or Spanish type, cut | 2 to 3 months | 1 month |
| Fresh poultry | Chicken or turkey, whole | 1 to 2 days | 1 year |
| | Chicken or turkey, pieces | 1 to 2 days | 9 months |
| Fin fish | Fatty fish (bluefish, catfish, mackerel, mullet, salmon, tuna, etc.) | 1 to 3 days | 2 to 3 months |
| | Lean fish (cod, flounder, haddock, halibut, sole, etc.) | 1 to 3 days | 6 to 8 months |
| | Lean fish (pollock, ocean perch, rockfish, sea trout) | 1 to 3 days | 4 to 8 months |

| FOOD | TYPE | REFRIGERATOR (40°F/4°C OR BELOW) | FREEZER (0°F/−18°C OR BELOW) |
| --- | --- | --- | --- |
| Shellfish | Fresh crab meat | 2 to 4 days | 2 to 4 months |
| | Fresh lobster | 2 to 4 days | 2 to 4 months |
| | Live crab, lobster | 1 day | Not recommended |
| | Live clams, mussels, oysters and scallops | 5 to 10 days | Not recommended |
| | Shrimp, crayfish | 3 to 5 days | 6 to 18 months |
| | Shucked clams, mussels, oysters and scallops | 3 to 10 days | 3 to 4 months |
| | Squid | 1 to 3 days | 6 to 18 months |
| Eggs | Raw eggs in shell | 3 to 5 weeks | Do not freeze in shell. Beat yolks and whites together, then freeze. |
| | Raw egg whites and yolks<br><br>Note: yolks do not freeze well | 2 to 4 days | 1 year |
| | Raw egg accidentally frozen in shell<br><br>Note: toss any frozen eggs with a broken shell | Use immediately after thawing | Keep frozen, then refrigerate to thaw |
| | Hard-cooked eggs | 1 week | Do not freeze |
| | Egg substitutes, liquid, unopened | 1 week | Do not freeze |
| | Egg substitutes, liquid, opened | 3 days | Do not freeze |
| | Egg substitutes, frozen, unopened | After thawing, 1 week or refer to “use by” date | 1 year |

| FOOD | TYPE | REFRIGERATOR (40°F/4°C OR BELOW) | FREEZER (0°F/−18°C OR BELOW) |
|---|---|---|---|
| Eggs *(continued)* | Egg substitutes, frozen, opened | After thawing, 3 to 4 days or refer to "use by" date | Do not freeze |
| | Casseroles with eggs | After baking, 3 to 4 days | After baking, 2 to 3 months |
| | Eggnog, commercial | 3 to 5 days | 6 months |
| | Eggnog, homemade | 2 to 4 days | Do not freeze |
| | Pies: pumpkin or pecan | After baking, 3 to 4 days | After baking, 1 to 2 months |
| | Pies: custard or chiffon | After baking, 3 to 4 days | Do not freeze |
| | Quiche with filling | After baking, 3 to 5 days | After baking, 2 to 3 months |
| Soups and stews | Vegetable or meat added | 3 to 4 days | 2 to 3 months |
| Leftovers | Cooked meat or poultry | 3 to 4 days | 2 to 6 months |
| | Chicken nuggets or patties | 3 to 4 days | 1 to 3 months |
| | Pizza | 3 to 4 days | 1 to 2 months |

## References

U.S. Department of Agriculture. Safe Minimum Internal Temperature Chart. Food Safety and Inspection Service. Updated April 14, 2025. Accessed November 15, 2025. https://www.fsis.usda.gov/food-safety/safe-food-handling-and-preparation/food-safety-basics/safe-temperature-chart.

U.S. Department of Health and Human Services. Food Safety Charts: Cold Food Storage Chart. FoodSafety.gov. Updated September 19, 2023a. Accessed November 17, 2025. https://www.foodsafety.gov/food-safety-charts/cold-food-storage-charts.

U.S. Department of Health and Human Services. Keep Food Safe: 4 Steps to Food Safety. FoodSafety.gov. Updated September 18, 2023b. Accessed November 17, 2025. https://www.foodsafety.gov/keep-food-safe/4-steps-to-food-safety.

## CHAPTER 10

# RECIPES AND INTERPRETING THE NUTRITION SCALE

*Our recipes were created to help folks living with Parkinson's eat in a way that supports health, energy and day-to-day function, without sacrificing enjoyment.*

Parkinson's disease touches every part of life, and food is no exception. Our recipes were created with a simple but powerful goal: to help folks living with Parkinson's eat in a way that supports health, energy and day-to-day function, without sacrificing enjoyment. We chose these recipes deliberately, not as rigid rules. We chose them as practical options to fit real lives.

You will find a wide variety of nourishing breakfasts, satisfying lunches, balanced dinners, smart snacks and even desserts that respect both health and pleasure. Each recipe was selected with Parkinson's in mind, focusing on whole foods, nutrient density and approaches that are realistic for individuals and families navigating the complexities of this disease. Many of the recipes are Mediterranean diet focused, as this approach has been linked to better brain health.

To make this book as useful as possible, we have added clear guidance using icons at the top of every recipe. We also mark the type of Parkinson's diet each recipe supports, the amount of fiber, the amount of protein and the level of complexity required for meal preparation. These unique Parkinson's nutrition scales are not provided as "academic extras." They are powerful tools to help you make informed choices based on your symptoms, schedule and energy level. Whether you are managing constipation, balancing protein intake around your medications or simply seeking a healthy stress-free meal, these markers were designed for you.

Parkinson's is a whole-body disease, and what you eat influences far more than just your weight and your cholesterol. The foods we choose shape inflammation, energy, mood and the microbiome. Your microbiome communicates directly with your brain. We believe that paying attention to diet and gut health can improve Parkinson's symptoms and can enhance overall well-being. These recipes, and this cookbook, are an invitation to view meals not as another burden of Parkinson's, but rather as a daily opportunity to support your body, your brain and your quality of life. There is a path to health with Parkinson's disease and that path includes both your diet and your lifestyle.

## INTERPRETING THE PARKINSON'S NUTRITION SCALES

The **protein scale** designates if a recipe is low, moderate or high in protein. People that experience medication–diet interactions may need lower-protein meals, while a person with unintentional weight loss may need higher-protein meals and snacks.

LOW MODERATE HIGH

**PROTEIN**

The **fiber scale** designates if a recipe is low, moderate or high in fiber. People that experience gastroparesis or gastrointestinal upset may need lower-fiber meals, while a person with constipation may need higher-fiber meals.

LOW MODERATE HIGH

**FIBER**

The **skill level scale** designates if a recipe is low, moderate or high in difficulty. This scale takes into account the time needed to prepare the recipe as well as the simplicity of the cooking methods and skills involved in combining ingredients. For people looking for low-effort meals or those with limited mobility or energy, the low-skill recipes are most fitting. For people looking to enhance their cooking skills and culinary experience, the high-skill recipes are most fitting.

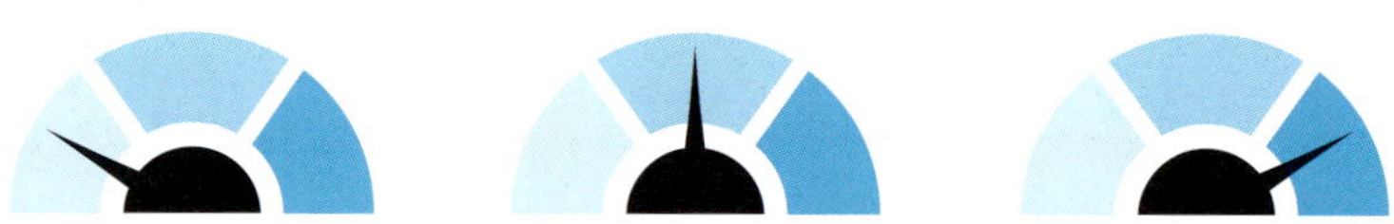

LOW MODERATE HIGH

**SKILL**

## INTERPRETING THE ICONS

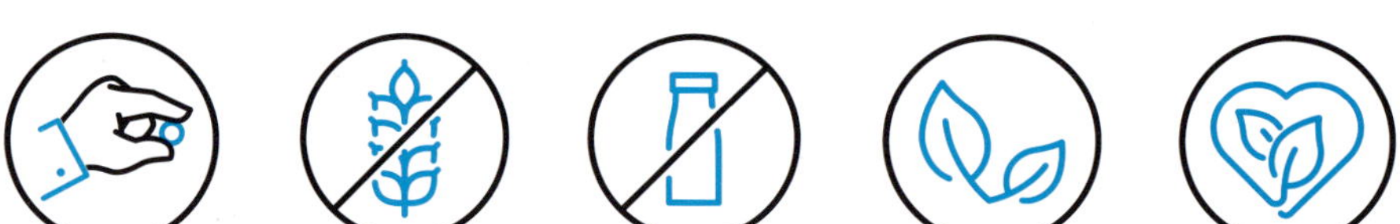

Finger Food Gluten-Free Dairy-Free Vegetarian Vegan

# LIST OF RECIPES

CHAPTER 11

# BREAKFAST

# Strawberry Breakfast Smoothies

- DYSPHAGIA-FRIENDLY
- HIGH CALORIE
- MEDITERRANEAN DIET
- MIND DIET

**MAKES 2 SERVINGS**

**SERVING SIZE: 2 CUPS (500 ML)**

A refreshing and balanced breakfast. A smoothie might be easier for people struggling with a decreased appetite. The chia seeds, oats, strawberries and banana provide a good source of fiber to start your day.

**Not all oats are gluten-free so be careful to buy oats that are labeled as "gluten-free" if you require that option.*

## TIP

For a vegan version, substitute plant-based dairy alternatives for the yogurt and milk.

- Blender

| | | |
|---|---|---|
| 1/4 cup | quick-cooking rolled oats | 60 mL |
| 1 tbsp | chia seeds | 15 mL |
| 2 cups | frozen strawberries | 500 mL |
| 1 cup | plain yogurt | 250 mL |
| 1 cup | milk | 250 mL |
| 1 | ripe banana | 1 |
| 2 tbsp | strawberry jam | 30 mL |

1. In a blender, place oats and chia seeds; blend until finely ground. Add strawberries, yogurt, milk, banana and jam; blend until smooth.

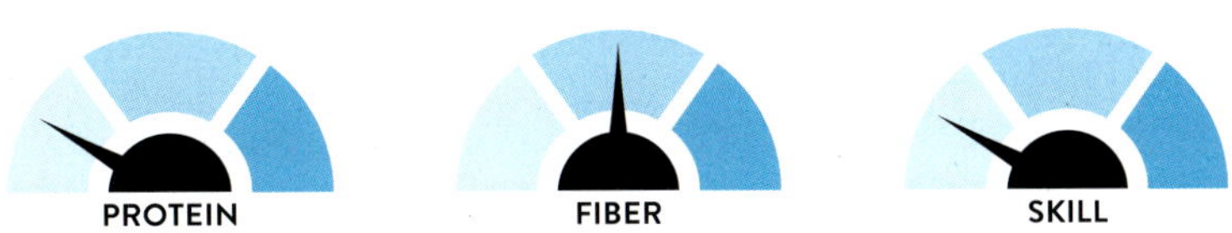


**NUTRIENTS PER SERVING**

| | | | | | |
|---|---|---|---|---|---|
| Calories | 320 kcal | Sodium | 160 mg | Vitamin D | 3 mcg |
| Fat | 3.5 g | Carbohydrate | 61 g | Calcium | 398 mg |
| Saturated fat | 0.5 g | Fiber | 7 g | Iron | 1 mg |
| Cholesterol | 5 mg | Protein | 13 g | Potassium | 839 mg |

# Silky Chocolate Breakfast Shake

- DYSPHAGIA-FRIENDLY
- HIGH CALORIE
- MEDITERRANEAN DIET

**MAKES 2 SERVINGS**

**SERVING SIZE:**
**¾ CUP (175 ML)**

This simple shake is full of healthy fats, which makes it a higher-calorie option for people trying to maintain weight. Use more frozen banana for a thicker consistency or add more milk for a thinner shake.

### TIP

The riper the banana, the sweeter the shake will be. For a lower-fat shake, opt for nonfat or low-fat chocolate milk.

- Blender

| | | |
|---|---|---|
| 2 | frozen bananas | 2 |
| 2 cups | chocolate milk | 500 mL |
| ½ | avocado | ½ |

1. Combine the bananas, chocolate milk and avocado in blender and blend until smooth.
2. Divide the shake evenly among glasses and enjoy!

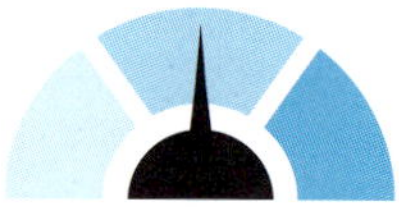

**NUTRIENTS PER SERVING**

| | | | | | |
|---|---|---|---|---|---|
| Calories | 320 kcal | Sodium | 160 mg | Vitamin D | 3 mcg |
| Fat | 9 g | Carbohydrate | 55 g | Calcium | 328 mg |
| Saturated fat | 2 g | Fiber | 6 g | Iron | 1 mg |
| Cholesterol | 15 mg | Protein | 10 g | Potassium | 1040 mg |

# Maple Berry Compote with Yogurt

- DYSPHAGIA-FRIENDLY
- HIGH CALORIE

**MAKES 1 SERVING**

This simple breakfast combines the rich protein from Greek yogurt with fiber-rich berries and oats, supporting a healthy metabolism and gut microbiome.

**Not all oats in granola are gluten-free so be careful to buy granola that is labeled as "gluten-free" if you require that option.*

### TIPS

This also makes a not-too-sweet dessert. Try topping it with crumbled cookies or toasted almonds in place of the granola.

If you prefer, you can use vanilla- or fruit-flavored Greek yogurt in place of the plain yogurt.

- 16-oz (500 mL) mug

| | | |
|---|---|---|
| **1 cup** | **frozen mixed berries** | **250 mL** |
| **6 tsp** | **pure maple syrup, divided** | **30 mL** |
| **1/8 tsp** | **ground cinnamon** | **0.5 mL** |
| **1/2 cup** | **plain Greek yogurt** | **125 mL** |
| **2 tbsp** | **granola (optional)** | **30 mL** |

1. In the mug, combine berries, 4 tsp (20 mL) maple syrup and cinnamon.
2. Microwave on High for 1 minute. Stir with a fork, then coarsely mash the berries. Microwave on High for 60 to 90 seconds or until bubbling at edges. Let cool for 1 to 2 minutes.
3. Spoon in the yogurt, sprinkle with granola (if using) and drizzle with remaining syrup.

### BLACKBERRY COMPOTE WITH CARDAMOM YOGURT

Use frozen blackberries in place of the mixed berries and replace the maple syrup with liquid honey. Omit the cinnamon and mix a pinch of ground cardamom into the yogurt.

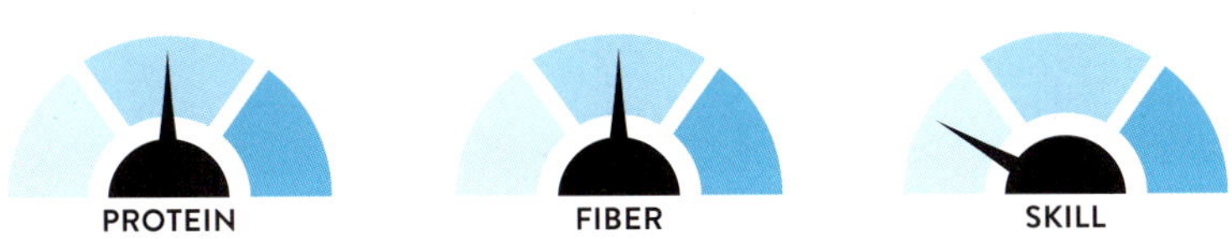


**NUTRIENTS PER SERVING**

| | | | | | |
|---|---|---|---|---|---|
| Calories | 316 kcal | Sodium | 55 mg | Vitamin D | 50 mcg |
| Fat | 11 g | Carbohydrate | 48 g | Calcium | 223 mg |
| Saturated fat | 7 g | Fiber | 5 g | Iron | 1 mg |
| Cholesterol | 38 mg | Protein | 9 g | Potassium | 1 mg |

# Hot Millet Amaranth Cereal

- DYSPHAGIA-FRIENDLY
- LOW CARBOHYDRATE
- MEDITERRANEAN DIET
- MIND DIET

**MAKES 6 SERVINGS**

A simple blend of whole grains that provide essential B vitamins and fiber. Dress this cereal up however you would like by adding nuts, seeds, dried fruit, and honey or brown sugar. Pair with your favorite milk or protein shake to support muscle health.

### TIP

For best results, toast the millet and amaranth before cooking. Stir the grains in a dry skillet over medium heat until they crackle and release their aroma, about 5 minutes.

| | | |
|---|---|---|
| 2½ cups | water | 625 mL |
| ½ cup | millet, toasted (see Tip, left) | 125 mL |
| ½ cup | amaranth, toasted (see Tip, left) | 125 mL |
| | Honey, pure maple syrup or raw cane sugar | |
| | Milk or non-dairy alternative | |
| | Dried cranberries, cherries or raisins (optional) | |
| | Toasted chopped nuts (optional) | |

1. In a saucepan over medium heat, bring water to a boil. Add millet and amaranth in a steady stream, stirring constantly. Return to a boil. Reduce heat to low. Cover and simmer until grains are tender and liquid is absorbed, about 25 minutes.
2. Serve hot, sweetened to taste and with milk or non-dairy alternative. Sprinkle with cranberries and nuts, if using.

### SLOW COOKER METHOD

Use a small (3½ quart/3.3 L) lightly greased slow cooker. Combine ingredients in slow cooker, adding ½ cup (125 mL) additional water to mixture. Place a clean tea towel folded in half (so you will have two layers) over top of the slow cooker to absorb moisture. Cover and cook on Low for 8 hours or overnight, or on High for 4 hours.

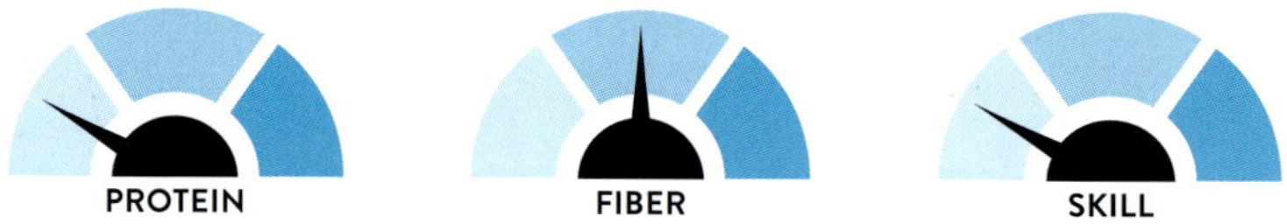


**NUTRIENTS PER SERVING**

| | | | | | |
|---|---|---|---|---|---|
| Calories | 200 kcal | Sodium | 40 mg | Vitamin D | 0 mcg |
| Fat | 8 g | Carbohydrate | 28 g | Calcium | 66 mg |
| Saturated fat | 1 g | Fiber | 4 g | Iron | 2 mg |
| Cholesterol | 0 mg | Protein | 5 g | Potassium | 171 mg |

# Overnight Applesauce Oats

- MEDITERRANEAN DIET
- MIND DIET

**MAKES 2 SERVINGS**

**SERVING SIZE: ABOUT 1 CUP (250 ML)**

This 3-ingredient breakfast is the perfect option for busy mornings. Make ahead the night before. You can change it up by adding your favorite fruit. Stir in some Greek yogurt or your favorite protein powder for even more protein.

**Not all oats are gluten-free so be careful to buy oats that are labeled as "gluten-free" if you require that option.*

- Two 8-oz (250 mL) glass jars with lids

| | | |
|---|---|---|
| 1 cup | large-flake (old-fashioned) rolled oats | 250 mL |
| $1\frac{1}{3}$ cups | milk | 325 mL |
| 1 cup | unsweetened applesauce | 250 mL |

1. Add half the oats, half the milk and half the applesauce to each jar and stir to combine. Cover with the lid and place in the refrigerator overnight.
2. In the morning, remove the jars from the refrigerator and stir to recombine. If you prefer warm oats, remove the lid and place one jar in the microwave for 2 minutes.

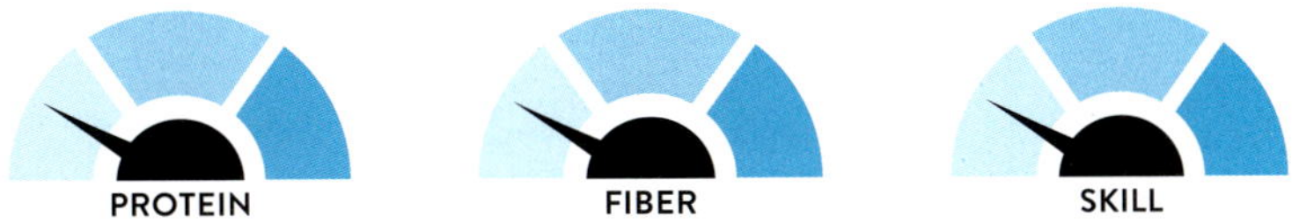


**NUTRIENTS PER SERVING**

| | | | | | |
|---|---|---|---|---|---|
| Calories | 289 kcal | Sodium | 74 mg | Vitamin D | 0 mcg |
| Fat | 5 g | Carbohydrate | 53 mg | Calcium | 223 mg |
| Saturated fat | 2 g | Fiber | 4 g | Iron | 2 mg |
| Cholesterol | 8 mg | Protein | 11 g | Potassium | 510 mg |

# Açai Superfood Bowl

- DYSPHAGIA-FRIENDLY
- MEDITERRANEAN DIET
- MIND DIET

**MAKES 2 SERVINGS**

Açai is a type of berry that is full of vitamins, minerals and antioxidants. Blended with other high-fiber fruits, it makes for a refreshing breakfast option. The use of a blender for this recipe means most people can easily prepare this nutrient-dense meal.

## TIPS

Using frozen berries helps make the mixture thick and rich. You can substitute an equal quantity of frozen strawberries or raspberries for the blueberries.

Açai powder is available in well-stocked supermarkets, natural food stores and online specialty stores.

- Blender

| | | |
|---|---|---|
| 1 cup | freshly squeezed orange juice | 250 mL |
| ½ cup | frozen blueberries (see Tips, left) | 125 mL |
| ¼ cup | chia seeds | 60 mL |
| 2 tbsp | freeze-dried açai powder | 30 mL |
| ¼ tsp | alcohol-free organic vanilla extract | 1 mL |
| ½ cup | chopped mango | 125 mL |
| ¼ cup | each chopped apple, raspberries and hulled strawberries | 60 mL |
| 2 tbsp | raw shelled hemp seeds | 30 mL |
| 2 tbsp | raw cashews | 30 mL |

1. In blender, at high speed, blend juice, blueberries, chia, açai powder and vanilla until smooth. Transfer to serving bowls. Top with remaining ingredients. Serve immediately.

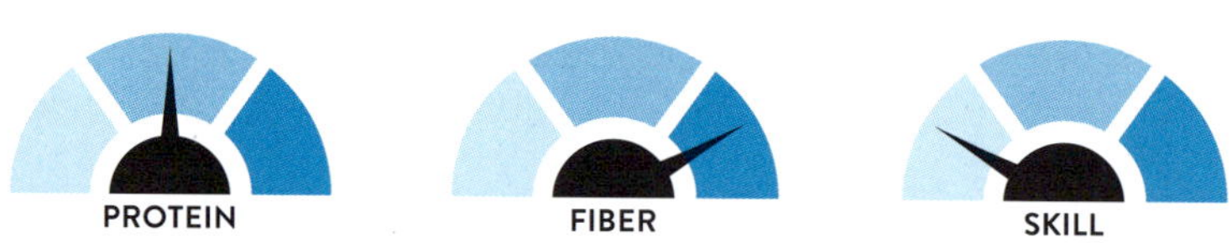


**NUTRIENTS PER SERVING**

| | | | | | |
|---|---|---|---|---|---|
| Calories | 420 kcal | Sodium | 95 mg | Vitamin D | 0 mcg |
| Fat | 21 g | Carbohydrate | 51 g | Calcium | 209 mg |
| Saturated fat | 2 g | Fiber | 19 g | Iron | 4 mg |
| Cholesterol | 0 mg | Protein | 12 g | Potassium | 566 mg |

# Morning Energy Bars

- HIGH CALORIE
- LOW CARBOHYDRATE
- MEDITERRANEAN DIET
- MIND DIET

**MAKES 8 BARS**

**SERVING SIZE: 1 BAR**

This is a great make-ahead breakfast option for busy mornings! These chocolatey breakfast bars can be taken on the go and may be easier to eat for those with self-feeding difficulty. They could also be served as a high-calorie, high-protein snack for people that need help maintaining weight.

| | | |
|---|---|---|
| 1¼ cups | almond flour | 310 mL |
| ¾ cup | chocolate protein powder | 175 mL |
| ¼ cup | unsweetened shredded coconut | 60 mL |
| ⅓ cup | ground flax seeds | 75 mL |
| ¾ cup | peanut butter | 175 mL |
| 3 tbsp | honey | 45 mL |
| ½ cup | unsweetened plain almond milk | 125 mL |
| 1 tsp | vanilla extract | 5 mL |
| ½ cup | mini chocolate chips | 125 mL |

1. In a medium bowl, combine almond flour, protein powder, coconut and ground flax seeds.
2. In a medium microwave-safe bowl, combine peanut butter and honey. Microwave on High for 30 seconds or until melted; stir until smooth. Add almond milk and vanilla; stir until milk is well incorporated. Pour peanut butter mixture over almond flour mixture and stir until well combined and crumbly.
3. Sprinkle half the chocolate chips in the bottom of a 9-inch (23 cm) square baking dish. Crumble dough evenly into pan and sprinkle remaining chocolate chips on top. Press mixture firmly into pan. Transfer to refrigerator to chill for 30 minutes.
4. Remove from refrigerator and cut into 8 bars. Serve immediately.

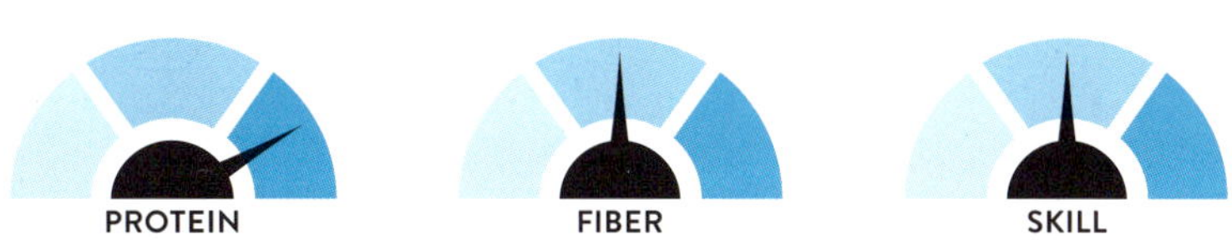


**NUTRIENTS PER SERVING**

| | | | | | |
|---|---|---|---|---|---|
| Calories | 450 kcal | Sodium | 300 mg | Vitamin D | 0 mcg |
| Fat | 30 g | Carbohydrate | 28 g | Calcium | 121 mg |
| Saturated fat | 7 g | Fiber | 5 g | Iron | 5 mg |
| Cholesterol | 0 mg | Protein | 23 g | Potassium | 471 mg |

# Zucchini Muffins

- DYSPHAGIA-FRIENDLY
- LOW PROTEIN

**MAKES 12 MUFFINS**

**SERVING SIZE: 1 MUFFIN**

A great way to sneak in extra vegetables! These muffins can be made ahead of time and reheated for a quick breakfast on the go. Opt for whole wheat flour and extra-virgin olive oil for a Mediterranean-forward variation.

- Preheat oven to 375°F (190°C)
- Food processor
- 12-cup muffin pan, coated with nonstick cooking spray or lined with paper liners

| | | |
|---|---|---|
| 1 | medium unpeeled zucchini | 1 |
| ½ cup | canola oil | 125 mL |
| ¾ cup | packed brown sugar | 175 mL |
| 2 | large eggs | 2 |
| 1 tsp | vanilla extract | 5 mL |
| 1 cup | all-purpose flour | 250 mL |
| ½ cup | whole wheat flour | 125 mL |
| 2 tsp | ground cinnamon | 10 mL |
| ½ tsp | baking soda | 2 mL |
| ½ tsp | baking powder | 2 mL |
| ½ tsp | salt | 2 mL |
| ¼ tsp | ground nutmeg | 1 mL |

1. In a food processor fitted with a grater attachment, grate zucchini. Measure out 1¾ cups (425 mL) grated zucchini and transfer to a small bowl. (Any leftover zucchini can be used in a salad, added to soup or sautéed.) In the same food processor bowl, without washing it and using the multipurpose blade, add oil, brown sugar, eggs and vanilla; process for 5 seconds.
2. Remove lid and add flours, cinnamon, baking soda, baking powder, salt and nutmeg. Pulse 10 times, or until ingredients are mostly blended. Scrape down the inside of the bowl and add zucchini; pulse 5 to 6 times, until just blended. Do not overmix.

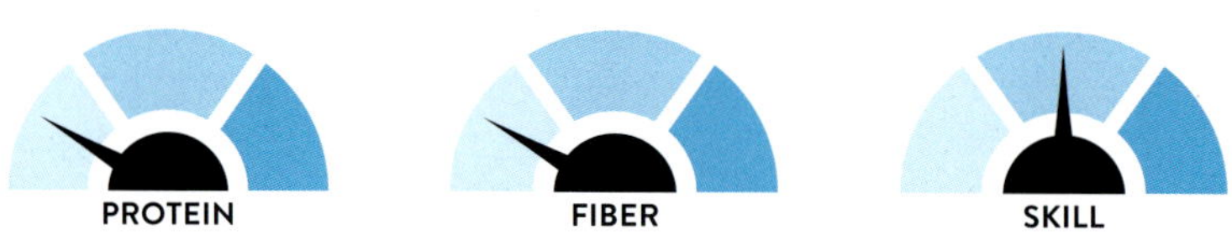


**NUTRIENTS PER SERVING**

| | | | | | |
|---|---|---|---|---|---|
| Calories | 250 kcal | Sodium | 290 mg | Vitamin D | 0 mcg |
| Fat | 13 g | Carbohydrate | 30 g | Calcium | 88 mg |
| Saturated fat | 3 g | Fiber | 1 g | Iron | 1 mg |
| Cholesterol | 35 mg | Protein | 3 g | Potassium | 98 mg |

### TIP

Muffins are best fresh, but they will keep in an airtight container at room temperature for 2 days. Muffins can also be frozen in an airtight container for up to 2 months.

3. Divide the batter into prepared muffin pan. Bake 20 to 25 minutes, or until an inserted toothpick comes out clean. Cool in pan for 5 minutes, then transfer muffins onto a rack to finish cooling.

## STREUSEL-TOPPED VARIATION

| | | |
|---|---|---|
| **¼ cup** | **all-purpose flour** | **60 mL** |
| **3 tbsp** | **packed brown sugar** | **45 mL** |
| **¼ tsp** | **ground cinnamon** | **1 mL** |
| **2 tbsp** | **butter, melted** | **30 mL** |

In a small bowl, combine flour, brown sugar, cinnamon and butter until crumbly mixture forms. Sprinkle on top of muffins just before baking.

# Chocolate Chip Walnut Muffins

- HIGH CALORIE
- MEDITERRANEAN DIET
- MIND DIET

**MAKES 12 MUFFINS**

**SERVING SIZE: 1 MUFFIN**

The walnuts in these muffins are a great source of unsaturated healthy fats that support the immune system and overall health. Pair these muffins with your favorite fruit and a glass of milk.

- Preheat oven to 350°F (180°C)
- 12-cup muffin pan, coated with nonstick cooking spray

| | | |
|---|---|---|
| 1½ cups | unbleached all-purpose flour | 375 mL |
| 1 cup | 100% whole wheat flour | 250 mL |
| 2 tsp | baking powder | 10 mL |
| ½ tsp | baking soda | 2 mL |
| ½ tsp | salt | 2 mL |
| 1 cup | low-fat (1%) milk | 250 mL |
| ½ cup | plain nonfat Greek yogurt | 125 mL |
| ½ cup | packed light brown sugar | 125 mL |
| ¼ cup | canola oil | 60 mL |
| ¼ cup | unsalted butter, melted | 60 mL |
| 1 | large egg, beaten | 1 |
| 1 tsp | vanilla extract | 5 mL |
| ¾ cup | raw or unsalted dry-roasted walnuts, coarsely chopped | 175 mL |
| ¾ cup | semisweet or dark chocolate chips | 175 mL |

1. In a medium bowl, sift together the all-purpose flour, whole wheat flour, baking powder, baking soda and salt. In a separate medium bowl, whisk together the milk, yogurt, brown sugar, oil, butter, egg and vanilla.
2. Gently fold the dry mixture into the wet mixture with as few strokes as possible until moistened. Do not overmix. Add the walnuts and chocolate chips and fold until just combined.

PROTEIN

FIBER

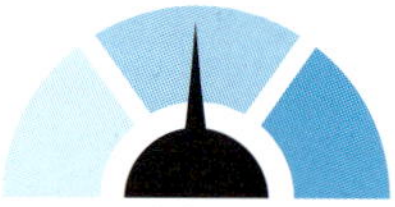

SKILL

**NUTRIENTS PER SERVING**

| | | | | | |
|---|---|---|---|---|---|
| Calories | 350 kcal | Sodium | 140 mg | Vitamin D | 0 mcg |
| Fat | 19 g | Carbohydrate | 39 g | Calcium | 167 mg |
| Saturated fat | 7 g | Fiber | 3 g | Iron | 2 mg |
| Cholesterol | 25 mg | Protein | 7 g | Potassium | 231 mg |

**TIP**

Walnuts are a great source of omega-3 fatty acids. However, you can add variety by incorporating your favorite nuts or seeds. Substitute chopped pecans for another tasty variation.

3. Divide the batter evenly among the 12 muffin cups. Tap the muffin pan several times on the counter to get rid of any air bubbles.

4. Bake in the center of the oven until a tester inserted into two muffins comes out clean, 18 to 20 minutes. Remove from the oven and let cool for 2 to 3 minutes in the pan. Remove the muffins from pan and finish cooling on a wire rack for 10 minutes.

5. Serve immediately or store at room temperature in a sealable container for up to 5 days.

# Ricotta Toast

**MAKES 2 SERVINGS**

**SERVING SIZE: 1 TOAST**

A quick and easy breakfast, this toast may be easier to handle for those that have difficulty using utensils.

### TIPS

To lighten up the dish, choose part-skim ricotta cheese.

To increase the fiber, choose a whole wheat brioche or other whole wheat bread.

| | | |
|---|---|---|
| ¼ cup | ricotta cheese | 60 mL |
| 2 | slices brioche bread, toasted | 2 |
| 2 tbsp | blueberry jam | 30 mL |

1. Spread 2 tbsp (30 mL) of the ricotta cheese on each slice of toast. Spoon 1 tbsp (15 mL) of the blueberry jam into the center of the ricotta cheese. Serve immediately.

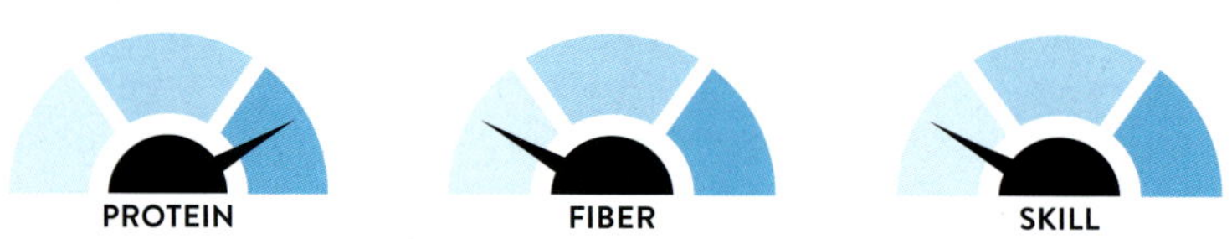


**NUTRIENTS PER SERVING**

| | | | | | |
|---|---|---|---|---|---|
| Calories | 280 kcal | Sodium | 370 mg | Vitamin D | 0 mcg |
| Fat | 1.5 g | Carbohydrate | 45 g | Calcium | 320 mg |
| Saturated fat | 0 g | Fiber | 1 g | Iron | 1 mg |
| Cholesterol | 30 mg | Protein | 17 g | Potassium | 35 mg |

# Avocado Toast with Tomato

- MEDITERRANEAN DIET
- MIND DIET

**MAKES 2 SERVINGS**

**SERVING SIZE: 1 TOAST**

Avocado is a great source of unsaturated fats and fiber. This minimal-ingredient breakfast helps support energy levels and gut health.

### TIPS

To increase the fiber, use 100% whole wheat or whole rye bread.

Strawberries can be swapped for tomatoes in many recipes, including this one, to give a sweet take on the dish.

| | | |
|---|---|---|
| ½ | **avocado** | ½ |
| 2 | **slices white bread, toasted** | 2 |
| | **Salt and ground black pepper** | |
| 6 | **cherry tomatoes, halved** | 6 |

1. Using a knife, slice the avocado flesh and spoon it out of the peel onto the bread. Use a fork to mash the avocado onto the toasts.
2. Season with salt and pepper to taste.
3. Top with halved cherry tomatoes.

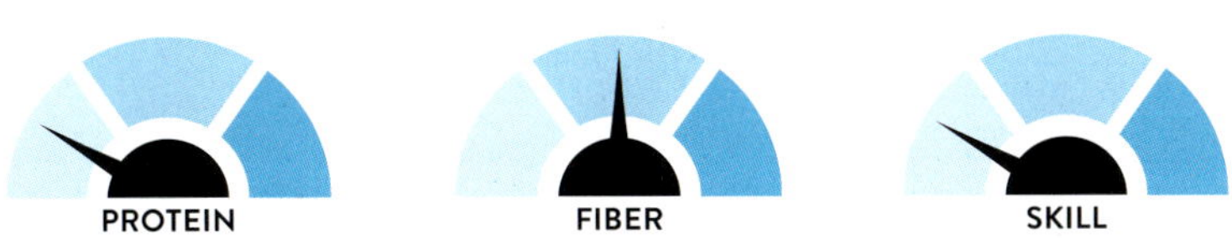


**NUTRIENTS PER SERVING**

| | | | | | |
|---|---|---|---|---|---|
| Calories | 210 kcal | Sodium | 210 mg | Vitamin D | 0 mcg |
| Fat | 8 g | Carbohydrate | 32 g | Calcium | 45 mg |
| Saturated fat | 1 g | Fiber | 4 g | Iron | 2 mg |
| Cholesterol | 0 mg | Protein | 4 g | Potassium | 358 mg |

# Almond Butter and Pear Toast

- HIGH CALORIE
- MEDITERRANEAN DIET
- MIND DIET

**MAKES 2 SERVINGS**

**SERVING SIZE: 1 TOAST**

This is a great high-calorie, high-fiber breakfast that does not require the use of utensils. Change it up by switching out the pear slices for your favorite fruit.

### TIP

To find out if a pear is ready to eat, check the neck. Use your thumb and forefinger to gently press on the neck of the pear. If it gives slightly, it's ripe!

| | | |
|---|---|---|
| 1/4 cup | almond butter | 60 mL |
| 2 tbsp | water | 30 mL |
| 1 tsp | pure maple syrup | 5 mL |
| 1/4 tsp | ground cinnamon | 1 mL |
| 2 | slices 100% whole wheat bread, toasted | 2 |
| 1/2 | pear, cored and thinly sliced | 1/2 |
| 2 tsp | chopped unsalted roasted almonds | 10 mL |

1. In a small saucepan, add the almond butter, water, maple syrup and cinnamon and place over high heat. Bring the mixture to a boil while whisking constantly. Reduce the heat to low and continue whisking until the almond butter mixture softens, about 1 minute. Remove the saucepan from the heat and let cool for 5 minutes.
2. On each slice of bread, spread about half of the almond butter mixture and top with half of the pear slices. Sprinkle each slice with half of the chopped almonds. Serve immediately.

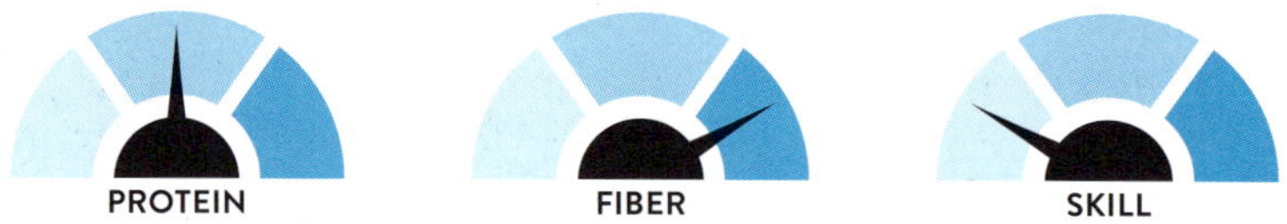


**NUTRIENTS PER SERVING**

| | | | | | |
|---|---|---|---|---|---|
| Calories | 350 kcal | Sodium | 290 mg | Vitamin D | 0 mcg |
| Fat | 21 g | Carbohydrate | 35 g | Calcium | 177 mg |
| Saturated fat | 3 g | Fiber | 9 g | Iron | 2 mg |
| Cholesterol | 0 mg | Protein | 12 g | Potassium | 431 mg |

# Breakfast Casserole

- DYSPHAGIA-FRIENDLY
- GLUTEN-FREE
- HIGH CALORIE

**MAKES 10 SERVINGS**

This is a great recipe to make the night before because it needs to sit for at least six hours before baking. In the morning, bake and eat. Simple!

**TIP**
Fresh fruit salad makes a lovely side dish with breakfast casseroles.

- 13- by 9-inch (33 by 23 cm) glass baking dish, greased

| | | |
|---|---|---|
| 1½ lbs | spicy pork sausage (bulk or removed from casings) | 750 g |
| 6 | eggs, lightly beaten | 6 |
| 2 lbs | frozen hash brown potatoes | 1 kg |
| 1 cup | minced onion | 250 mL |
| 2 cups | milk | 500 mL |
| 4 cups | shredded Colby-Jack or Cheddar cheese (about 1 lb/500 g), divided | 1 L |
| ½ tsp | salt | 2 mL |
| | Salsa | |

1. In a large nonstick skillet over medium-high heat, cook sausage, breaking it up with the back of a spoon, for 8 to 10 minutes or until no longer pink. Drain off fat. Let cool for 5 minutes.
2. In a large bowl, combine sausage, eggs, hash browns, onion, milk, 3 cups (750 mL) of the cheese and salt. Pour into prepared baking dish. Top with the remaining cheese. Cover and refrigerate for at least 6 hours or overnight.
3. Preheat oven to 350°F (180°C).
4. Uncover baking dish. Bake for 50 to 55 minutes or until a knife inserted in the center comes out clean. Cover and let stand for 10 minutes. Cut into squares and serve immediately with salsa.

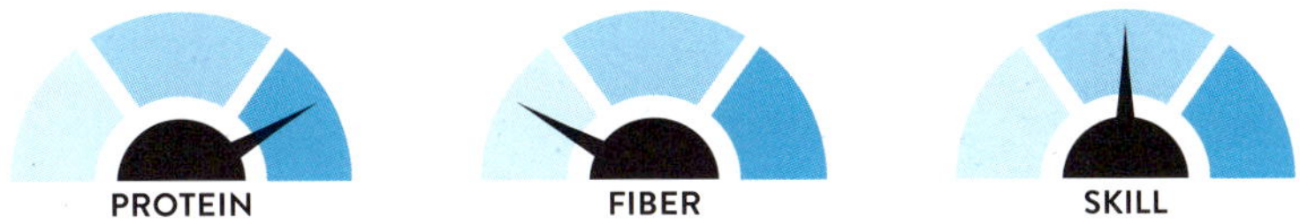


**NUTRIENTS PER SERVING**

| | | | | | |
|---|---|---|---|---|---|
| Calories | 720 kcal | Sodium | 1,820 mg | Vitamin D | 1 mcg |
| Fat | 51 g | Carbohydrate | 35 g | Calcium | 438 mg |
| Saturated fat | 18 g | Fiber | 0 g | Iron | 2 mg |
| Cholesterol | 190 mg | Protein | 29 g | Potassium | 463 mg |

# Sheet-Pan Breakfast Bagel Sandwiches

HIGH CALORIE

**MAKES 4 SERVINGS**

**SERVING SIZE: 1 BAGEL SANDWICH**

A complete meal! To keep the sandwich together while eating it, try using sandwich picks. Add vegetables such as tomato, onion and spinach for a fiber-rich variation.

- Preheat oven to 425°F (220°C)
- Rimmed sheet pan

| | | |
|---|---|---|
| 4 | large eggs | 4 |
| | Everything bagel spice blend | |
| 4 | bagels, split | 4 |
| | Butter for spreading on bagels | |
| 4 | thin slices smoked deli ham (about 6 oz/175 g total) | 4 |
| 4 | slices sharp (old) Cheddar cheese (about 6 oz/175 g total) | 4 |
| 1 | green onion, chopped | 1 |
| 1 | tomato, thinly sliced | 1 |
| 1 | avocado, thinly sliced | 1 |

1. Line one-third of rimmed sheet pan with foil, and fold edges up to create a lip all around to help keep the eggs together while they bake. Spray foil with nonstick cooking spray. Gently crack the eggs onto the foil, then sprinkle with a bit of the spice blend. Bake for 3 minutes.

2. Meanwhile, butter the bagels. After the eggs have baked for 3 minutes, arrange bagels on pan, butter side up, on the empty side of the sheet pan. Place a slice of ham on 4 of the bagel halves, followed by a slice of cheese and a sprinkle of green onion. Return pan to oven and bake another 2 to 3 minutes or until eggs are cooked to desired doneness and cheese is melted.

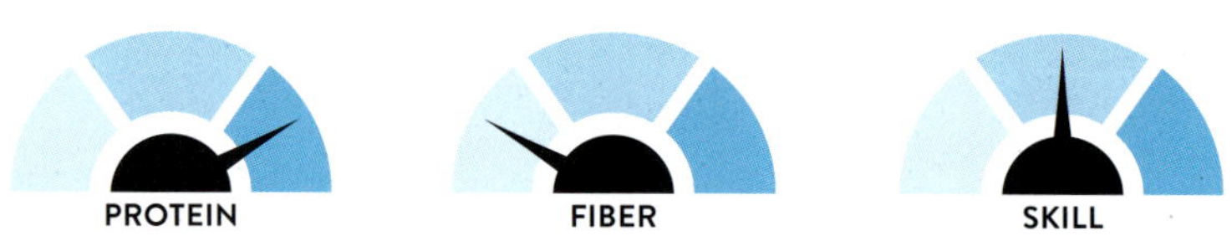


**NUTRIENTS PER SERVING**

| | | | | | |
|---|---|---|---|---|---|
| Calories | 660 kcal | Sodium | 1,410 mg | Vitamin D | 1 mcg |
| Fat | 29 g | Carbohydrate | 64 g | Calcium | 453 mg |
| Saturated fat | 12 g | Fiber | 3 g | Iron | 6 mg |
| Cholesterol | 250 mg | Protein | 26 g | Potassium | 441 mg |

**TIP**
Instead of Cheddar cheese slices, try with mozzarella, Havarti or jalapeño Jack cheese.

3. To assemble, place one egg on the ham and bagel half, along with a slice of tomato and avocado. Top with the other half of the bagel. Serve hot.

# Chorizo Tempeh Breakfast Wraps

- HIGH CALORIE
- MEDITERRANEAN DIET

**MAKES 4 SERVINGS**

**SERVING SIZE: 1 WRAP**

This quick sheet-pan meal saves time and energy. It's a great use of plant-based protein, and the addition of sweet potato, onion and kale helps pack in extra nutrients. Make this gluten-free by using corn tortillas instead of flour tortillas.

- Preheat the oven to 400°F (200°C)
- Large rimmed baking sheet, lined with parchment paper

| | | |
|---|---|---|
| 1½ cups | peeled and cubed sweet potato (about 1 small) | 375 mL |
| ½ | onion, sliced | ½ |
| 2 tbsp | vegetable oil, divided | 30 mL |
| ½ tsp | salt | 2 mL |
| 12 oz | tempeh, roughly chopped | 375 g |
| 1 | red bell pepper, sliced | 1 |
| 1 tbsp | nutritional yeast | 15 mL |
| 1 tsp | chili powder | 5 mL |
| 1 tsp | ground cumin | 5 mL |
| ¼ tsp | garlic powder | 1 mL |
| 2 cups | coarsely chopped, ribs-removed kale | 500 mL |
| 4 | 12 inch (30 cm) flour tortillas | 4 |
| ½ cup | tomato salsa | 125 mL |

1. Place the sweet potato, onion, 1 tbsp (15 mL) oil and salt in a large bowl; toss to coat. Spread onto the prepared baking sheet in an even layer (reserve the bowl) and bake in the preheated oven for 10 minutes or until the onion is starting to brown.

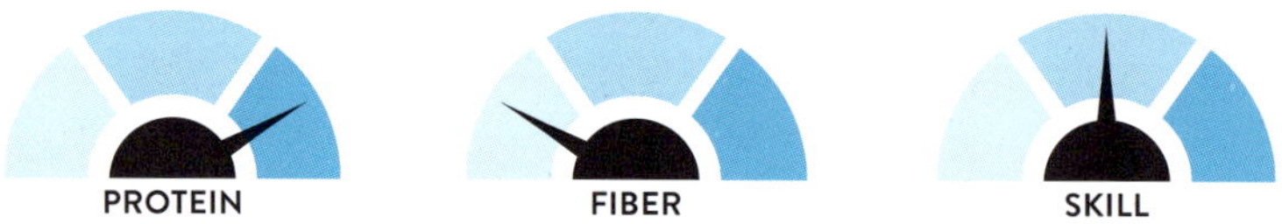


**NUTRIENTS PER SERVING**

| | | | | | |
|---|---|---|---|---|---|
| Calories | 490 kcal | Sodium | 970 mg | Vitamin D | 0 mg |
| Fat | 23 g | Carbohydrate | 50 g | Calcium | 255 mg |
| Saturated fat | 5 g | Fiber | 3 g | Iron | 5 mg |
| Cholesterol | 0 mg | Protein | 26 g | Potassium | 540 mg |

### TIP

These wraps are great to make ahead, but the directions differ slightly from the recipe.

**To freeze:** Let the filling cool completely. Assemble through Step 3, but do not add salsa. Wrap tightly in plastic wrap and store in the freezer for up to 3 months.

**To reheat from frozen in the microwave:** Remove plastic, then wrap tortilla in a damp paper towel. Place on a plate and microwave on High for 2 to 3 minutes, until heated through.

**To reheat from frozen in the oven:** Preheat the oven to 375°F (190°C). Remove plastic and place tortilla on a baking sheet. Bake in the oven for 20 minutes or until heated through.

2. Meanwhile, add the tempeh, red pepper, remaining 1 tbsp (15 mL) oil, nutritional yeast, chili powder, cumin and garlic powder to the reserved bowl; toss to coat. Transfer to the baking sheet and stir gently to combine.
3. Bake for about 15 minutes, until the sweet potato is fork-tender and the tempeh is golden. Add the kale and bake for 2 more minutes, until the kale is slightly wilted.
4. Divide the mixture among the tortillas and top evenly with salsa. Fold in the sides and roll each tortilla up from the bottom, like a burrito. Serve.

# Garden Vegetable Frittata

- DYSPHAGIA-FRIENDLY
- KETOGENIC DIET
- LOW CARBOHYDRATE
- MEDITERRANEAN DIET

**MAKES 6 SERVINGS**

A great way to incorporate more vegetables at the start of your day!

- Preheat oven to 350°F (180°C)
- 11- by 7-inch (28 by 18 cm) glass baking dish, greased

| | | |
|---|---|---|
| 1 lb | asparagus, trimmed and cut into 1-inch (2.5 cm) pieces | 500 g |
| | Ice water | |
| 1 tbsp | olive oil | 15 mL |
| 4 oz | mushrooms, sliced | 125 g |
| 1 | clove garlic, minced | 1 |
| 1 | shallot, minced | 1 |
| 1 | small zucchini, cut in half lengthwise and thinly sliced | 1 |
| 6 | eggs | 6 |
| 1/3 cup | milk | 75 mL |
| 1 tbsp | chopped fresh chives | 15 mL |
| 1 tsp | salt | 5 mL |
| 1/2 tsp | ground black pepper | 2 mL |
| 1/8 tsp | ground nutmeg | 0.5 mL |
| 2 | tomatoes, thinly sliced | 2 |
| 1/4 cup | freshly grated Parmesan cheese | 60 mL |

1. In a large saucepan of boiling water, blanch asparagus for 1 to 2 minutes. Immediately plunge into ice water; let stand until chilled. Drain and place in prepared baking dish.
2. In a skillet, heat oil over medium heat. Sauté mushrooms for about 10 minutes or until tender. Add garlic and shallot; sauté for 2 minutes. Spread over asparagus. Arrange zucchini on top.

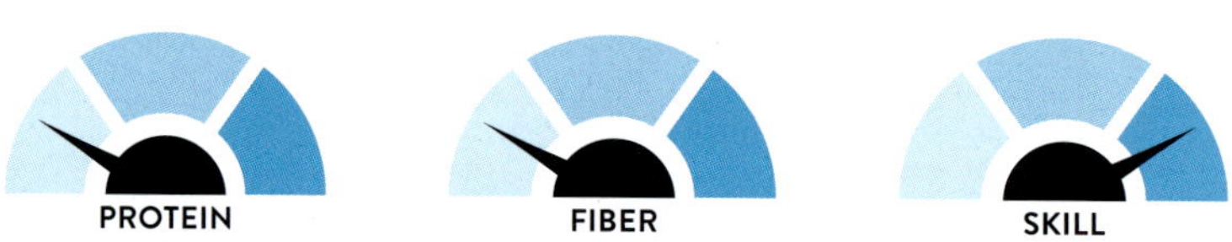


**NUTRIENTS PER SERVING**

| | | | | | |
|---|---|---|---|---|---|
| Calories | 130 kcal | Sodium | 510 mg | Vitamin D | 1 mcg |
| Fat | 8 g | Carbohydrate | 7 g | Calcium | 106 mg |
| Saturated fat | 2.5 g | Fiber | 2 g | Iron | 3 mg |
| Cholesterol | 170 mg | Protein | 9 g | Potassium | 397 mg |

**TIP**

Shocking vegetables in ice water stops the cooking process after blanching and sets the color, so you will have brightly colored vegetables even after baking.

3. In a large bowl, whisk eggs until blended. Whisk in milk, chives, salt, pepper and nutmeg. Pour evenly over vegetable mixture. Arrange tomatoes on top. Sprinkle evenly with cheese.

4. Bake in preheated oven for 40 to 45 minutes or until set.

# Artichoke Quiche

- DYSPHAGIA-FRIENDLY
- KETOGENIC DIET
- LOW CARBOHYDRATE
- MEDITERRANEAN DIET
- MIND DIET

**MAKES 8 SERVINGS**

**SERVING SIZE: 1 SLICE**

A quiche is a great way to feed many or have leftovers for the days ahead. This quiche is full of vegetables, including spinach, which is a key part of the MIND diet. Spinach is full of folate and fiber. Opt for low-fat cheese and whole wheat bread crumbs for a more Mediterranean-forward breakfast.

## TIPS

As the quiche bakes, you may need to cover the edges of the crust with foil to prevent excess browning.

Squeeze thawed and drained spinach several times to remove excess moisture.

- Preheat oven to 425°F (220°C)

| | | |
|---|---|---|
| 1 | 9-inch (23 cm) unbaked pie shell | 1 |
| 6 | eggs | 6 |
| 1 | package (10 oz/300 g) frozen chopped spinach, thawed and squeezed dry | 1 |
| 1 | can (14 oz/398 mL) artichoke hearts, drained and chopped | 1 |
| 1 | small onion, finely chopped | 1 |
| 1 | clove garlic, minced | 1 |
| 2 cups | shredded Cheddar cheese | 500 mL |
| 1/2 cup | chopped mushrooms | 125 mL |
| 1/4 cup | dry bread crumbs | 60 mL |
| 1/2 tsp | salt | 2 mL |
| 1/4 tsp | ground black pepper | 1 mL |
| 1/4 tsp | dried oregano | 1 mL |
| 1/4 tsp | hot pepper sauce | 1 mL |

1. Prick pie shell all over with a fork. Bake in preheated oven for 5 to 10 minutes or until lightly browned. Let cool slightly. Reduce oven temperature to 350°F (180°C).
2. In a large bowl, whisk eggs until blended. Stir in spinach, artichokes, onion, garlic, cheese, mushrooms, bread crumbs, salt, pepper, oregano and hot pepper sauce. Pour into pie crust.
3. Bake for 55 to 60 minutes or until a knife inserted in the center comes out clean.

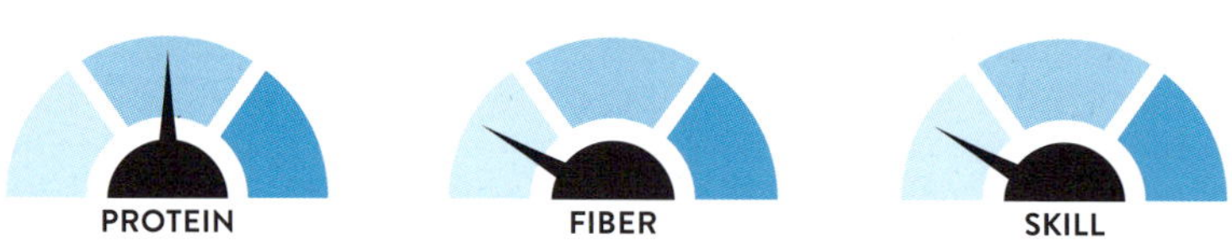


**NUTRIENTS PER SERVING**

| | | | | | |
|---|---|---|---|---|---|
| Calories | 220 kcal | Sodium | 450 mg | Vitamin D | 1 mcg |
| Fat | 14 g | Carbohydrate | 10 g | Calcium | 269 mg |
| Saturated fat | 7 g | Fiber | 2 g | Iron | 2 mg |
| Cholesterol | 150 mg | Protein | 13 g | Potassium | 351 mg |

# Pumpkin Oat Pancakes

- MEDITERRANEAN DIET
- MIND DIET

**MAKES 4 SERVINGS**

**SERVING SIZE: 2 PANCAKES**

The oats in this recipe provide a sustainable source of energy to start your morning. Pair with a side of Greek yogurt or scrambled eggs for additional protein.

**Not all oats are gluten-free so be careful to buy oats that are labeled as "gluten-free" if you require that option.*

### TIP

Choose canned 100% pumpkin made of only pumpkin and skip the canned pumpkin pie purée, which contains added sugar.

- Blender

| | | |
|---|---|---|
| 1½ cups | canned 100% pumpkin (see Tip, left) | 375 mL |
| 1½ cups | large-flake (old-fashioned) rolled oats | 375 mL |
| ¼ cup | liquid honey | 60 mL |
| ¾ cup | water | 175 mL |
| 3 tbsp | olive oil, divided | 45 mL |

1. Place the pumpkin, oats, honey, water and 1 tbsp (15 mL) of the oil in a blender and blend until smooth. Spoon into a medium bowl.
2. Heat 1 tbsp (15 mL) of the oil in a large skillet over medium heat.
3. When the oil is shimmering, scoop ¼ cup (60 mL) of the pancake mixture onto the heated skillet. Repeat to make a total of 4 pancakes in the skillet. Cook until the pancakes begin to brown, about 3 minutes, and then flip and press down gently with the back of a spatula. Cook an additional 2 to 3 minutes on the other side. Transfer cooked pancakes to a clean plate and cover with foil to keep warm.
4. Add another 1 tbsp (15 mL) of oil to the skillet to begin a new batch. Continue until all the pancakes are cooked. Serve warm.

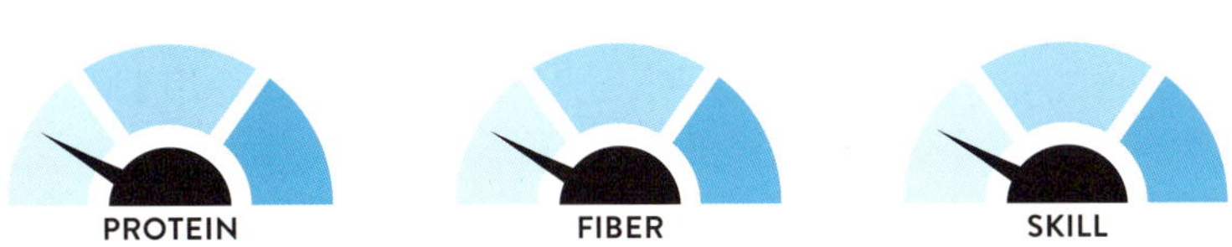


**NUTRIENTS PER SERVING**

| | | | | | |
|---|---|---|---|---|---|
| Calories | 250 kcal | Sodium | 10 mg | Vitamin D | 0 mcg |
| Fat | 12 g | Carbohydrate | 35 g | Calcium | 23 mg |
| Saturated fat | 1.5 g | Fiber | 2 g | Iron | 2 mg |
| Cholesterol | 0 mg | Protein | 3 g | Potassium | 70 mg |

# CHAPTER 12

# LUNCH

# Turkey Sausage Sandos

▸ HIGH CALORIE

**MAKES 4 SERVINGS**

**SERVING SIZE: 1 SANDWICH**

Instead of making a sandwich, the turkey sausage mixture could be served by itself or over rice for a more dysphagia-friendly option.

### TIP

You can substitute your favorite pork or plant-based sausages in this recipe too.

| | | |
|---|---|---|
| 1 tbsp | canola oil | 15 mL |
| 1 | small onion, chopped | 1 |
| 1 | small green bell pepper, chopped | 1 |
| 2 | cloves garlic, minced | 2 |
| 1 lb | mild Italian turkey sausages, casings removed | 454 g |
| 2 tsp | dried oregano | 10 mL |
| 1/4 tsp | hot pepper flakes | 1 mL |
| 1 | can (19 oz/540 mL) petite-cut stewed tomatoes | 1 |
| 2 tbsp | tomato paste | 30 mL |
| 2 tsp | Worcestershire sauce | 10 mL |
| 1/4 tsp | salt | 1 mL |
| 4 | Kaiser buns | 4 |
| 4 | slices provolone cheese | 4 |
| 1 cup | packed baby arugula | 250 mL |

1. In a large nonstick skillet, heat oil over medium heat and cook onion, green pepper and garlic for about 3 minutes or until softened. Add turkey sausage, oregano and hot pepper flakes and cook, breaking up with a wooden spoon, for about 5 minutes or until no longer pink.
2. Add tomatoes, tomato paste, Worcestershire sauce and salt. Simmer gently for 15 minutes or until thickened.
3. Open buns and place bottom half on each plate and spoon turkey mixture over top. Top with provolone and arugula. Sandwich with top bun to serve.

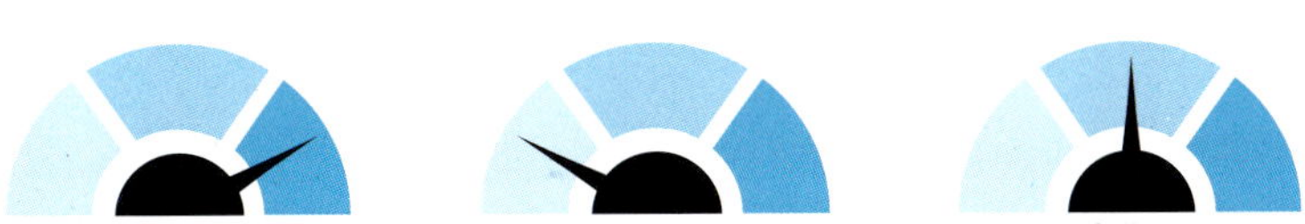

PROTEIN FIBER SKILL

**NUTRIENTS PER SERVING**

| | | | | | |
|---|---|---|---|---|---|
| Calories | 510 kcal | Sodium | 1,460 mg | Vitamin D | 0 mcg |
| Fat | 19 g | Carbohydrate | 50 g | Calcium | 239 mg |
| Saturated fat | 5 g | Fiber | 5 g | Iron | 5 mg |
| Cholesterol | 85 mg | Protein | 34 g | Potassium | 546 mg |

# Avocado Egg Salad–Stuffed Pita

▸ MEDITERRANEAN DIET

**MAKES 6 SERVINGS**

**SERVING SIZE: 1 STUFFED PITA**

This recipe is the perfect blend of healthy fats, fiber and protein, making it a quick and nutrient-dense lunch. Eat the pita as the recipe calls for or scoop up the avocado egg salad with whole wheat crackers. Avocados are a great source of unsaturated fats, fiber and potassium, and are a key part of the Mediterranean diet.

## TIP

I typically call for plum (Roma) tomatoes in sandwiches, as they don't have many seeds and aren't as juicy as other tomatoes, which keeps the bread from getting soggy.

| | | |
|---|---|---|
| 6 | large eggs | 6 |
| 2 | avocados, halved and pitted | 2 |
| 2 tbsp | light mayonnaise | 30 mL |
| 2 tbsp | plain nonfat Greek yogurt | 30 mL |
| 2 tbsp | chopped fresh dill | 30 mL |
| | Juice of $\frac{1}{2}$ lemon | |
| $\frac{1}{4}$ tsp | salt | 1 mL |
| $\frac{1}{8}$ tsp | ground black pepper | 0.5 mL |
| 6 | large whole wheat pitas | 6 |
| 6 | leaves lettuce, halved | 6 |
| 2 | plum (Roma) tomatoes, thinly sliced | 2 |

1. In a medium saucepan, cover the eggs with water. Place the saucepan over high heat and bring the water to a boil. Boil the eggs for 3 minutes, then remove from the heat, cover and let the eggs stand for 15 minutes. Drain the water, and run cold water over the eggs until they are completely cool, about 10 minutes. Peel the eggs and coarsely chop.
2. Place the chopped eggs in a medium bowl. Using a spoon, scoop the avocados out of their skins and add to the eggs. Using the back of a fork or a potato masher, mash the egg and avocado mixture. Add the mayonnaise, yogurt, dill, lemon juice, salt and pepper and stir until combined.
3. Cut 1 inch (2.5 cm) off the top of the pitas.
4. Stuff each of the pitas with an even amount of lettuce and tomatoes. Add about $\frac{1}{2}$ cup (125 mL) of the egg mixture. Serve immediately.

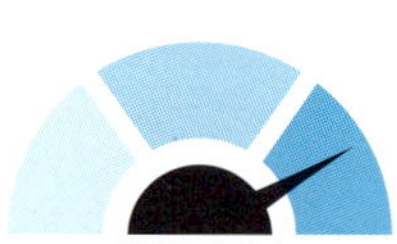


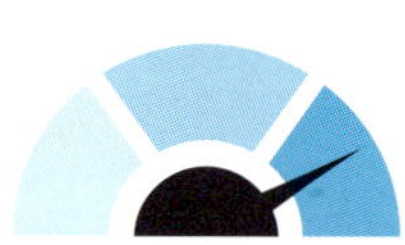


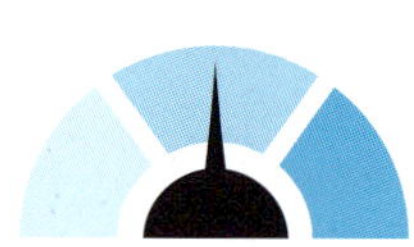


**NUTRIENTS PER SERVING**

| | | | | | |
|---|---|---|---|---|---|
| Calories | 410 kcal | Sodium | 550 mg | Vitamin D | 1 mcg |
| Fat | 19 g | Carbohydrate | 51 g | Calcium | 260 mg |
| Saturated fat | 4 g | Fiber | 15 g | Iron | 6 mg |
| Cholesterol | 185 mg | Protein | 20 g | Potassium | 1,503 mg |

# Avocado and White Bean Sandwich

▶ MEDITERRANEAN DIET

**MAKES 4 SANDWICHES**

**SERVING SIZE: 1 SANDWICH**

The combination of beans, avocado and whole wheat bread makes this recipe a great source of fiber. The avocado-white bean mixture on its own makes for a tasty snack for people with swallowing difficulty.

**TIP**

To make this recipe gluten-free, serve the avocado-bean mixture over a salad instead of on bread.

| | | |
|---|---|---|
| 1¾ cups | canned low-sodium cannellini (white kidney) or great northern beans, drained and rinsed | 425 mL |
| 2 | avocados, sliced | 2 |
| 1 tbsp | freshly squeezed lime juice | 15 mL |
| 1 | clove garlic, minced | 1 |
| 2 tbsp | chopped fresh parsley | 30 mL |
| 2 tbsp | chopped fresh cilantro | 30 mL |
| ¼ tsp | salt | 1 mL |
| ⅛ tsp | ground black pepper | 0.5 mL |
| ⅛ tsp | hot pepper flakes | 0.5 mL |
| 8 | slices 100% whole wheat bread, toasted | 8 |
| 4 oz | fire-roasted red bell peppers, cut into 4 equal slices | 125 g |
| 2 | mini cucumbers, thinly sliced | 2 |

1. In a large bowl, mash the beans with a fork or potato masher. Add the avocado and lime juice; mash until combined. Add the garlic, parsley, cilantro, salt, black pepper and hot pepper flakes; mash until combined.
2. Place 4 slices of toasted bread on a cutting board. On each piece, lay a slice of roasted red pepper and top with ½ cup (125 mL) avocado-bean mixture. Using the back of a spoon, press down lightly. Top with cucumber slices, dividing evenly, and a second piece of toast. Slice the sandwiches in half and serve immediately.

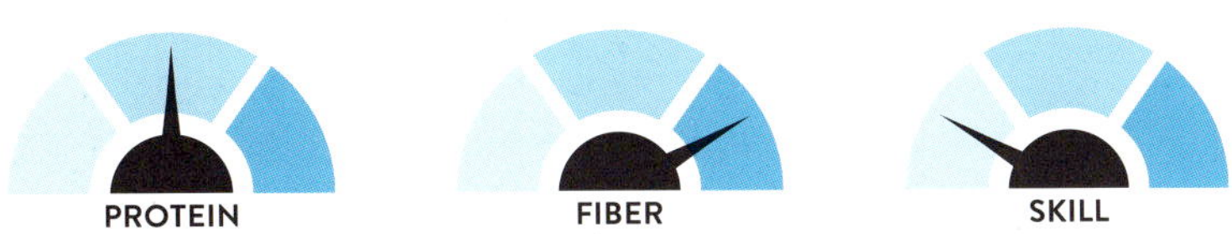


**NUTRIENTS PER SERVING**

| | | | | | |
|---|---|---|---|---|---|
| Calories | 400 kcal | Sodium | 560 mg | Vitamin D | 0 mcg |
| Fat | 17 g | Carbohydrate | 57 g | Calcium | 182 mg |
| Saturated fat | 2 g | Fiber | 19 g | Iron | 4 mg |
| Cholesterol | 0 mg | Protein | 14 g | Potassium | 1,149 mg |

# Veggie Chicken Salad Sandwich

▸ HIGH CALORIE

**MAKES 4 SANDWICHES**

**SERVING SIZE: 1 SANDWICH**

For people with swallowing difficulty, try serving the chicken salad on its own or with a side of cooked vegetables.

### TIP

A multifunctional veggie chopper can save many hours in the kitchen, not to mention that it creates evenly sized pieces. You can find many varieties online.

| | | |
|---|---|---|
| $\frac{1}{4}$ cup | light mayonnaise | 60 mL |
| 2 tbsp | plain nonfat Greek yogurt | 30 mL |
| 1 tsp | Dijon mustard | 5 mL |
| $\frac{1}{4}$ tsp | garlic powder | 1 mL |
| $\frac{1}{4}$ tsp | salt | 1 mL |
| $\frac{1}{8}$ tsp | ground black pepper | 0.5 mL |
| 1 | can (12.5 oz/354 g) chunk chicken breast, rinsed and drained, or equal amount of diced grilled boneless skinless breast | 1 |
| 2 | medium carrots, finely chopped | 2 |
| 2 | stalks celery, finely chopped | 2 |
| 1 | red bell pepper, finely chopped | 1 |
| 2 tbsp | chopped fresh parsley | 30 mL |
| 4 | leaves lettuce, halved | 4 |
| 8 | slices seedless rye bread | 8 |

1. In a small bowl, combine the mayonnaise, Greek yogurt, mustard, garlic powder, salt and black pepper.
2. In a medium bowl, combine the chicken, carrots, celery, red pepper and parsley. Add the mayonnaise mixture and stir to coat.
3. Place 2 lettuce leaf halves on each of 4 bread slices. Spread about $\frac{1}{2}$ cup (125 mL) chicken salad onto each lettuce stack and top with a second slice of bread. Cut in half; serve.

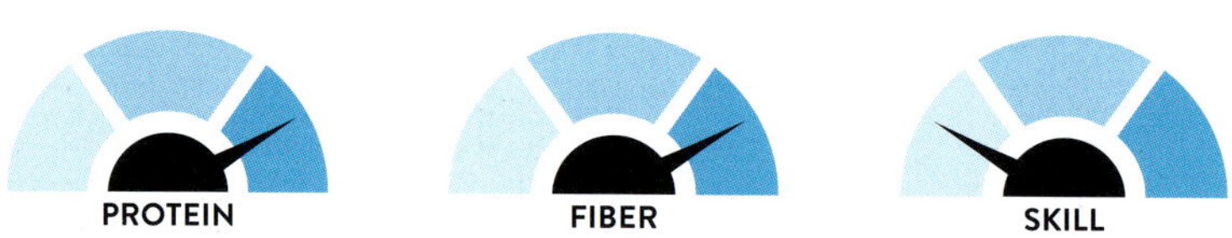


**NUTRIENTS PER SERVING**

| | | | | | |
|---|---|---|---|---|---|
| Calories | 480 kcal | Sodium | 1,060 mg | Vitamin D | 0 mcg |
| Fat | 14 g | Carbohydrate | 54 g | Calcium | 236 mg |
| Saturated fat | 3 g | Fiber | 8 g | Iron | 7 mg |
| Cholesterol | 85 mg | Protein | 40 g | Potassium | 1,440 mg |

# Orzo Salad with Red Bell Peppers and Mozzarella

- LOW CARBOHYDRATE
- MEDITERRANEAN DIET
- MIND DIET

**MAKES 6 SERVINGS**

**SERVING SIZE: ABOUT ¾ CUP (175 ML)**

A lower-calorie lunch option, this recipe provides just enough protein for those concerned about medication-dietary protein interactions. The dark leafy spinach, a staple in the MIND diet, is a great source of folate and iron.

### TIP

Swap the orzo for macaroni or another smaller-size pasta.

| | | |
|---|---|---|
| 6 oz | whole wheat orzo | 175 g |
| 5 tbsp | extra-virgin olive oil | 75 mL |
| 4 cups | baby spinach | 1 L |
| 1 cup | coarsely chopped fresh basil | 250 mL |
| 2 tbsp | red wine vinegar | 30 mL |
| 2 | cloves garlic, minced | 2 |
| ¼ tsp | salt | 1 mL |
| ⅛ tsp | ground black pepper | 0.5 mL |
| 1 | red bell pepper, diced | 1 |
| 4 oz | fresh mozzarella cheese, cut into ½-inch (1 cm) cubes | 125 g |
| 1 cup | halved grape tomatoes | 250 mL |

1. Fill a medium saucepan three-quarters full with water and bring to a boil over high heat. Add the orzo and cook until al dente, 7 to 8 minutes. Drain the orzo and let cool for 10 minutes.
2. In a large skillet, heat 1 tbsp (15 mL) of the oil over medium heat. Add the spinach and basil and cook until wilted, 3 to 4 minutes. Remove from the heat and set aside.
3. In a small bowl, whisk together the vinegar, garlic, salt and black pepper. Slowly drizzle in the remaining ¼ cup (60 mL) oil, continuously whisking, until incorporated.
4. In a large bowl, add the orzo and spinach mixture and toss to combine. Add the red pepper, cheese and tomatoes and toss to evenly incorporate. Drizzle the dressing onto the salad and toss to evenly coat.
5. Serve immediately or store in a covered container for up to 4 days in the refrigerator.

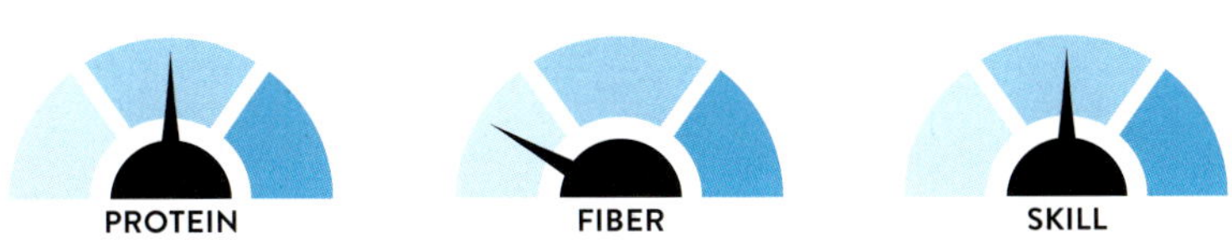


**NUTRIENTS PER SERVING**

| | | | | | |
|---|---|---|---|---|---|
| Calories | 290 kcal | Sodium | 135 mg | Vitamin D | 0 mcg |
| Fat | 15 g | Carbohydrate | 28 g | Calcium | 15 mg |
| Saturated fat | 4 g | Fiber | 2 g | Iron | 10 mg |
| Cholesterol | 10 mg | Protein | 11 g | Potassium | 2 mg |

# Falafel Salad with Tahini Dressing

▶ MEDITERRANEAN DIET

**MAKES 6 SERVINGS**

This higher-sodium vegan recipe is perfect for people looking to add salt to their diet to help manage orthostatic hypotension.

- Preheat oven to 400°F (200°C)
- Food processor
- Baking sheet, brushed with oil

### *Falafel*

| | | |
|---|---|---|
| 1 | can (19 oz/540 mL) chickpeas, rinsed and drained | 1 |
| 2 | shallots, coarsely chopped | 2 |
| ½ cup | coarsely chopped fresh parsley | 125 mL |
| 2 tbsp | cornstarch | 30 mL |
| 1 tbsp | za'atar spice mix | 15 mL |
| ½ tsp | salt | 2 mL |
| 2 tbsp | canola oil | 30 mL |

### *Dressing*

| | | |
|---|---|---|
| ⅓ cup | tahini | 75 mL |
| ¼ cup | freshly squeezed lemon juice | 60 mL |
| 2 tsp | pure maple syrup | 10 mL |
| ¼ tsp | garlic powder | 1 mL |
| ¾ tsp | salt | 3 mL |
| 3 tbsp | warm water | 45 mL |

### *Salad*

| | | |
|---|---|---|
| 8 cups | chopped lettuce (such as romaine or green leaf) | 2 L |
| 2 cups | halved grape tomatoes | 500 mL |
| 1 | English cucumber, sliced | 1 |
| ½ | red onion, thinly sliced | ½ |

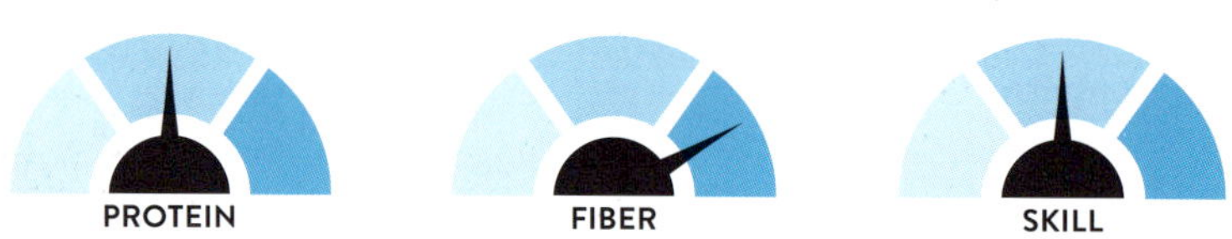


**NUTRIENTS PER SERVING**

| | | | | | |
|---|---|---|---|---|---|
| Calories | 340 kcal | Sodium | 730 mg | Vitamin D | 0 mcg |
| Fat | 14 g | Carbohydrate | 52 g | Calcium | 144 mg |
| Saturated fat | 2 g | Fiber | 12 g | Iron | 4 mg |
| Cholesterol | 0 mg | Protein | 12 g | Potassium | 953 mg |

## TIP

The dressing can be made and refrigerated for up to 5 days. Add water to thin dressing if needed.

1. **Make the falafel:** In a food processor, add chickpeas, shallots, parsley, cornstarch, za'atar and salt. Pulse to a crumbly consistency, until you can squeeze a ball that holds together and doesn't stick to your hands. (Scrape down sides of bowl as needed.) If mixture is too wet, add a little more cornstarch. Using a mini ice cream scoop or a tablespoon (15 mL) measure, scoop mixture (about 48 small balls) onto prepared baking sheet and slightly flatten each ball, then drizzle with oil. Bake 25 minutes until golden brown and crisp.
2. **Make the dressing:** Meanwhile, in a small bowl, whisk together tahini, lemon juice, maple syrup, garlic powder and salt; mixture will become very stiff. Add 3 tbsp (45 mL) water and continue whisking until mixture is well blended and creamy. Add more water, 1 tsp (5 mL) at a time, if you prefer the dressing to be thinner. Refrigerate until ready to use. Makes about 1 cup (250 mL).
3. **Assemble the salad:** Arrange lettuce, tomatoes, cucumber, red onion and falafel on a large platter or 6 individual plates. Drizzle with dressing just before serving.

# Mediterranean Bean Salad

▸ MEDITERRANEAN DIET

**MAKES 4 SERVINGS**

Quality ingredients, like a variety of beans, fresh vegetables, herbs and olive oil, make this Mediterranean-style salad full of antioxidants, fiber and unsaturated fats that are beneficial for brain health.

### TIP

**To soak the beans, chickpeas and cannellini beans:** Place in a bowl and cover with 8 cups (2 L) water. Cover and set aside for at least 6 hours or overnight (if overnight, refrigerate). Drain, discarding water.

| | | |
|---|---|---|
| 8 cups | water | 2 L |
| 1 cup | dried kidney beans, soaked (see Tip, at left) | 250 mL |
| 1/2 cup | dried chickpeas, soaked | 125 mL |
| 1/2 cup | dried cannellini (white kidney) beans, soaked | 125 mL |
| 1 tsp | fine sea salt, divided | 5 mL |
| 1/2 cup | chopped red bell pepper | 125 mL |
| 1/2 cup | chopped seeded peeled cucumber | 125 mL |
| 1/4 cup | extra-virgin olive oil | 60 mL |
| 3 tbsp | red wine vinegar | 45 mL |
| 2 tsp | dried oregano | 10 mL |
| 1 tsp | raw agave nectar or pure maple syrup | 5 mL |

1. In a large saucepan, combine water, soaked kidney beans, chickpeas and cannellini beans and 1/2 tsp (2 mL) salt. Bring to a boil, reduce heat and simmer until tender, about 1 hour. Drain, discarding water. Let cool.
2. In a large bowl, combine cooked beans mixture, remaining 1/2 tsp (2 mL) salt, red pepper, cucumber, oil, vinegar, oregano and agave nectar; toss until well combined. Serve immediately or transfer to an airtight container and refrigerate for up to 5 days.

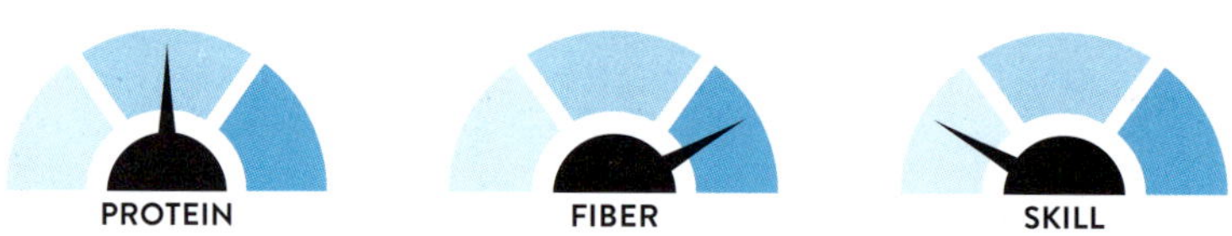


**NUTRIENTS PER SERVING**

| | | | | | |
|---|---|---|---|---|---|
| Calories | 330 kcal | Sodium | 820 mg | Vitamin D | 0 mcg |
| Fat | 17 g | Carbohydrate | 36 g | Calcium | 116 mg |
| Saturated fat | 3 g | Fiber | 9 g | Iron | 3 mg |
| Cholesterol | 0 mg | Protein | 11 g | Potassium | 603 mg |

# Sweet and Spicy Cauliflower and Chickpeas

- LOW CARBOHYDRATE
- MEDITERRANEAN DIET

**MAKES 4 SERVINGS**

Plant-based protein is a great way to incorporate protein for muscle health and fiber for gut health.

### TIP

There's no need to trim the leaves off the cauliflower, but do remove some of the tough stem. The leaves become wonderfully crisp in the oven.

- Preheat oven to 425°F (220°C)

| | | |
|---|---|---|
| 2 tbsp | canola oil, divided | 30 mL |
| 1 | (1 lb/500g) head cauliflower, cut into 4 wedges | 1 |
| ½ tsp | salt, divided | 2 mL |
| 1 | can (19 oz/540 mL) chickpeas, rinsed, drained and patted dry | 1 |
| 2 tsp | liquid honey | 10 mL |
| 2 tsp | ketchup | 10 mL |
| 2 tsp | soy sauce | 10 mL |
| 1½ tsp | chili garlic sauce | 7 mL |
| 1 tsp | cider vinegar | 5 mL |
| 2 tsp | toasted sesame seeds | 10 mL |
| 1 | green onion, thinly sliced | 1 |

1. In a heavy ovenproof skillet, heat 1 tbsp (15 mL) oil over medium-high heat. Place cauliflower wedges cut side down and sprinkle with half the salt. Cook cauliflower without moving it for 7 minutes or until golden brown on the bottom, then flip pieces over. Sprinkle chickpeas around the cauliflower, drizzle with remaining oil, then sprinkle with remaining salt. Place skillet in oven and bake 25 minutes or until the cauliflower is tender.
2. Meanwhile, in a small bowl, whisk together honey, ketchup, soy sauce, chili garlic sauce and vinegar.
3. Remove skillet from oven and transfer cauliflower and chickpeas to a serving plate. Drizzle half of the sauce over top. Sprinkle with sesame seeds and green onion and serve remaining sauce on the side for dipping.

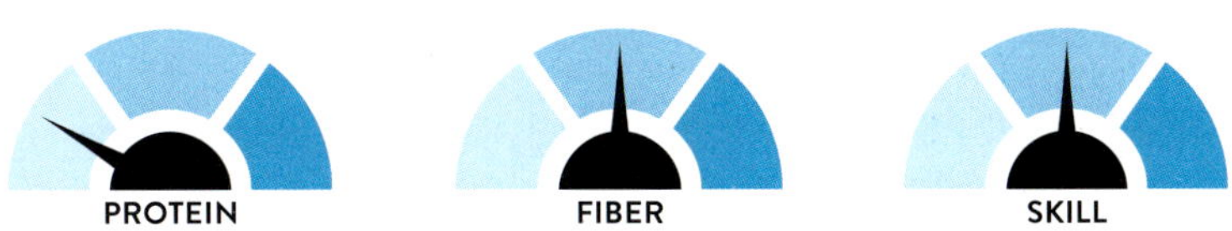


**NUTRIENTS PER SERVING**

| | | | | | |
|---|---|---|---|---|---|
| Calories | 210 kcal | Sodium | 730 mg | Vitamin D | 0 mcg |
| Fat | 9 g | Carbohydrate | 25 g | Calcium | 58 mg |
| Saturated fat | 0.5 g | Fiber | 7 g | Iron | 1 mg |
| Cholesterol | 0 mg | Protein | 8 g | Potassium | 94 mg |

# Brussels Sprouts, Kale and Farro Bowls

- HIGH CALORIE
- MEDITERRANEAN DIET
- MIND DIET

**MAKES 4 SERVINGS**

**SERVING SIZE: 1 BOWL**

Substitute quinoa or brown rice for farro for a gluten-free variation. Full of leafy greens and fiber for optimal energy throughout the day!

- Rimmed baking sheet, lined with parchment paper or a silicone mat
- Preheat the oven to 425°F (220°C)

| | | |
|---|---|---|
| 1 cup | farro | 250 mL |
| 2 cups | water | 500 mL |
| 1 cup | low-sodium vegetable broth | 250 mL |
| 1 lb | Brussels sprouts, halved | 500 g |
| 1 lb | butternut squash, cubed | 500 g |
| 3 tbsp | olive oil, divided | 45 mL |
| 2 tbsp | liquid honey | 30 mL |
| 1/4 tsp + 1/8 tsp | salt, divided | 1.5 mL |
| 6 cups | chopped kale | 1.5 L |
| 2 | medium carrots, shredded | 2 |
| 1/8 tsp | ground black pepper | 0.5 mL |
| 1/4 cup | chopped walnuts | 60 mL |
| 1/4 cup | crumbled goat cheese | 60 mL |

1. In a medium saucepan, combine the farro, water and vegetable broth; bring to a boil over high heat. Reduce heat to medium-low, cover and simmer until the farro is cooked through, about 30 minutes. Fluff with a fork and set aside to cool slightly.
2. In a large bowl, combine the Brussels sprouts, squash, 2 tbsp (30 mL) olive oil, honey and 1/4 tsp (1 mL) salt. Spread the mixture on the prepared baking sheet in a single layer.

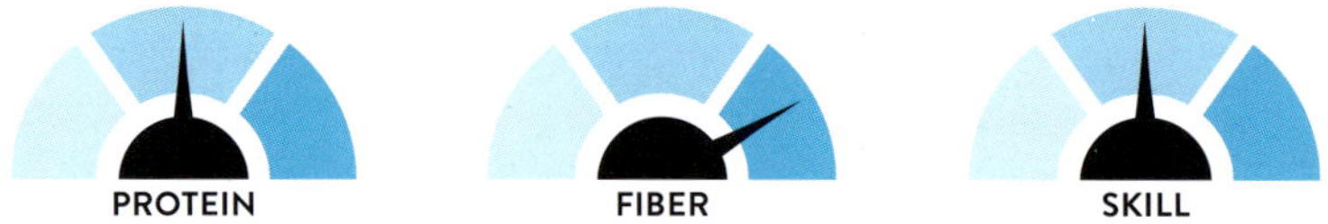


**NUTRIENTS PER SERVING**

| | | | | | |
|---|---|---|---|---|---|
| Calories | 490 kcal | Sodium | 360 mg | Vitamin D | 0 mcg |
| Fat | 20 g | Carbohydrate | 68 g | Calcium | 182 mg |
| Saturated fat | 4 g | Fiber | 13 g | Iron | 4 mg |
| Cholesterol | 10 mg | Protein | 16 g | Potassium | 1,250 mg |

**TIP**

The inclusion of a variety of vegetables and a whole grain make this recipe high in fiber. Fiber is important for feeding good bacteria in the gut. This can help balance the microbiome for those with dysbiosis or an imbalance of gut bacteria.

3. Roast the vegetables, turning halfway through, until they begin to brown, about 25 minutes. Remove the baking sheet from the oven and set aside to cool slightly, about 5 minutes.

4. In a large skillet, heat the remaining 1 tbsp (15 mL) olive oil over medium heat until shimmering. Add the kale, carrots, pepper and remaining ⅛ tsp (0.5 mL) salt; cook until the kale has wilted and carrots have softened, about 3 minutes.

5. In each of 4 bowls, arrange ½ cup (125 mL) cooked farro and 1½ cups (375 mL) roasted vegetable mixture side by side. Top with about ½ cup (125 mL) carrot-kale mixture. Sprinkle with 1 tbsp (15 mL) each of the walnuts and goat cheese. Serve warm.

# Speedy Vegetable Soup

▸ MEDITERRANEAN DIET
▸ MIND DIET

**MAKES 6 SERVINGS**

**SERVING SIZE:**
**1½ CUPS (375 ML)**

Quick, easy, stress-free and full of fiber, this classic blend of vegetables makes a nice light lunch. With a low amount of protein, it's ideal for people on a protein redistribution diet.

### TIP

Substitute the mixed vegetables with reduced-sodium canned or frozen vegetables such as green beans, asparagus, mushrooms, peas or carrots.

| | | |
|---|---|---|
| 2 tbsp | olive oil | 30 mL |
| 1 | medium onion, chopped | 1 |
| 2 | cloves garlic, minced | 2 |
| 4 cups | low-sodium vegetable broth | 1 L |
| 1 | can (28 oz/796 mL) crushed tomatoes | 1 |
| 3 cups | frozen mixed vegetables | 750 mL |
| 1 | can (5½ oz/156 mL) tomato paste | 1 |
| 1 tsp | dried Italian seasoning | 5 mL |
| ½ tsp | salt | 2 mL |
| ⅛ tsp | ground black pepper | 0.5 mL |
| 3 cups | lightly packed baby spinach | 750 mL |

1. In a large saucepan, heat the olive oil over medium heat until shimmering. Add the onion and garlic; cook, stirring occasionally, until the onion is translucent, about 3 minutes. Add the vegetable broth, crushed tomatoes, mixed vegetables, tomato paste, Italian seasoning, salt and pepper; increase the heat to high and bring to a boil. Reduce the heat to medium-low, cover and simmer, stirring occasionally, for 5 minutes. Add the spinach; cook, stirring occasionally, until wilted, about 2 minutes.

2. Ladle 1½ cups (375 mL) soup into each of 6 bowls. Serve warm.

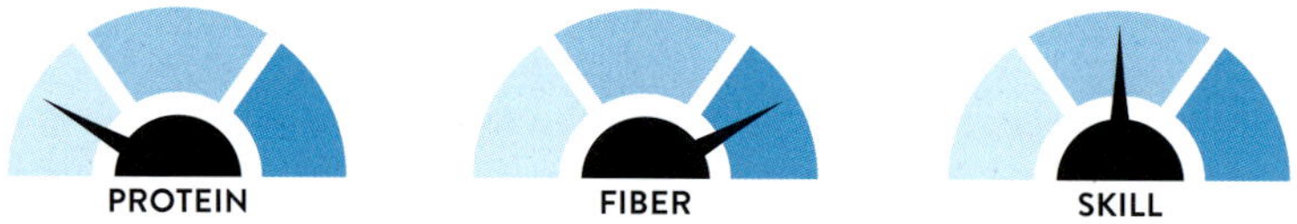


**NUTRIENTS PER SERVING**

| | | | | | |
|---|---|---|---|---|---|
| Calories | 210 kcal | Sodium | 730 mg | Vitamin D | 0 mcg |
| Fat | 5 g | Carbohydrate | 36 g | Calcium | 115 mg |
| Saturated fat | 0.5 g | Fiber | 10 g | Iron | 4 mg |
| Cholesterol | 0 mg | Protein | 9 g | Potassium | 634 mg |

# Hearty Root Vegetable and Chicken Soup

▸ MEDITERRANEAN DIET

**MAKES 4 SERVINGS**

**SERVING SIZE: 2 CUPS (500 ML)**

For anyone with swallowing difficulty: Once the soup is prepared, add a serving to a food processor to blend the ingredients into one consistency. This can be easier to eat than a soup with pieces of vegetables or other "chunky bits."

## TIP

To save time on a busy weeknight, chop all your vegetables and dice the rotisserie chicken in the morning before work or the night before. Place the ingredients in a covered container and use within 24 hours.

| | | |
|---|---|---|
| 2 tbsp | olive oil or canola oil | 30 mL |
| 1 | yellow onion, chopped | 1 |
| 1 | carrot, chopped | 1 |
| 1 | stalk celery, chopped | 1 |
| 1 | turnip, chopped | 1 |
| 2 | parsnips, chopped | 2 |
| 1 | can (14- to 19-oz/398 to 540 mL) reduced-sodium cannellini (white kidney) beans, drained and rinsed | 1 |
| 2 cups | chopped rotisserie chicken | 500 mL |
| 6 cups | reduced-sodium chicken broth | 1.5 L |
| 1 tbsp | mirin, dry sherry or sweet marsala wine | 15 mL |
| 2 | bay leaves | 2 |
| 1/4 tsp | salt | 1 mL |
| 1/4 tsp | ground black pepper | 1 mL |
| 2 cups | packed chopped kale or baby kale | 500 mL |

1. Heat the oil in a large saucepan over medium heat. When shimmering, add onion, carrot, celery, turnip and parsnips and sauté until onion is translucent and vegetables begin to soften, about 5 minutes.
2. Add beans and chicken and stir to combine. Add chicken broth, mirin, bay leaves, salt and pepper and stir to combine. Increase heat to high and bring to a boil, then reduce heat to medium-low, cover and simmer until the flavors combine and the vegetables are cooked, 20 minutes. Stir in kale and allow to wilt, 2 minutes. Discard bay leaves before serving.

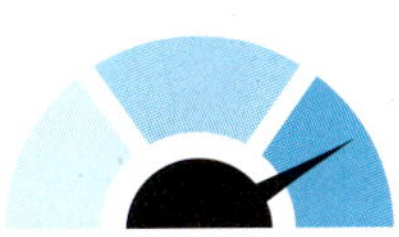

PROTEIN

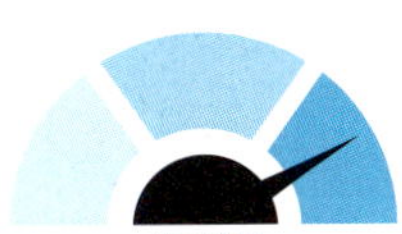

FIBER

SKILL

**NUTRIENTS PER SERVING**

| | | | | | |
|---|---|---|---|---|---|
| Calories | 450 kcal | Sodium | 860 mg | Vitamin D | 0 mcg |
| Fat | 20 g | Carbohydrate | 44 g | Calcium | 148 mg |
| Saturated fat | 4 g | Fiber | 11 g | Iron | 4 mg |
| Cholesterol | 75 mg | Protein | 28 g | Potassium | 1,122 mg |

# Kale Pesto Pasta

- HIGH CALORIE
- MEDITERRANEAN DIET

**MAKES 5 SERVINGS**

Choose a whole-grain pasta for a bit more fiber. Dark leafy kale provides essential fiber, folate and vitamin K!

**TIP**

Serve with additional Parmesan and black pepper on the side.

- **Food processor**

| | | |
|---|---|---|
| $\frac{3}{4}$ cup | toasted walnut pieces | 175 mL |
| 3 | cloves garlic | 3 |
| 1 tbsp | freshly squeezed lemon juice | 15 mL |
| $1\frac{1}{2}$ tsp | salt | 7 mL |
| $\frac{1}{2}$ tsp | ground black pepper | 2 mL |
| 3 cups | packed stemmed kale leaves | 750 mL |
| $\frac{3}{4}$ cup | grated Parmesan cheese | 175 mL |
| $\frac{1}{3}$ cup | extra-virgin olive oil | 75 mL |
| 12 oz | dried pasta, such as spaghetti | 375 g |

1. In the bowl of a food processor, add walnuts, garlic, lemon juice, salt and pepper; process until crumbly. Scrape down sides of bowl; add kale and cheese. With the machine running, slowly drizzle in oil. Process to desired consistency, scraping down sides if necessary.
2. Cook pasta for about 8 minutes or until al dente. Reserve $\frac{1}{2}$ cup (125 mL) of pasta cooking liquid, drain pasta and return to pot. Mix in enough pesto so it tastes good; add reserved cooking liquid if needed.

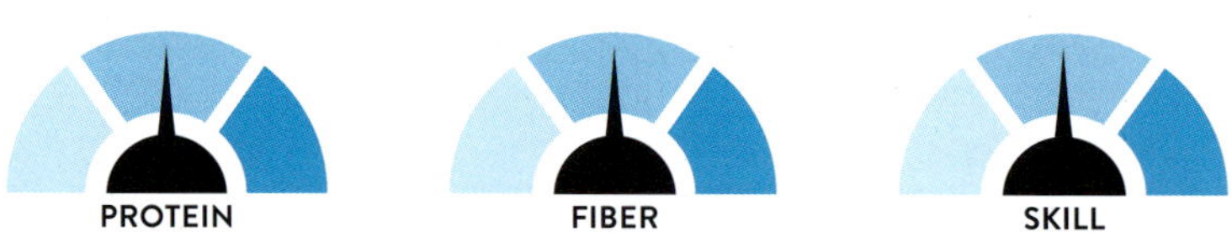


**NUTRIENTS PER SERVING**

| | | | | | |
|---|---|---|---|---|---|
| Calories | 580 kcal | Sodium | 920 mg | Vitamin D | 0 mcg |
| Fat | 31 g | Carbohydrate | 62 g | Calcium | 161 mg |
| Saturated fat | 5 g | Fiber | 4 g | Iron | 3 mg |
| Cholesterol | 10 mg | Protein | 17 g | Potassium | 336 mg |

# Cilantro Lime Chicken Tacos

▸ LOW CARBOHYDRATE

**MAKES 6 SERVINGS**

**SERVING SIZE: 2 TACOS**

Try topping your taco with fresh produce, such as chopped tomato, avocado and onion, for a burst of nutrients.

- Blender or food processor

| | | |
|---|---|---|
| $\frac{1}{3}$ cup | chicken broth | 75 mL |
| $2\frac{1}{2}$ tbsp | olive oil | 37 mL |
| 2 tbsp | minced garlic | 30 mL |
| 2 tsp | freshly squeezed lime juice | 10 mL |
| $\frac{1}{2}$ cup | freshly grated Parmesan cheese | 125 mL |
| 2 tbsp | sliced almonds (optional) | 30 mL |
| 1 tsp | salt | 5 mL |
| 1 cup | fresh cilantro leaves | 250 mL |
| 3 cups | shredded cooked chicken breast | 750 mL |
| 12 | 6 inch (15 cm) corn tortillas | 12 |
| $\frac{1}{2}$ cup | crumbled queso fresco (optional) | 125 mL |
| | Chopped fresh cilantro (optional) | |
| | Lime wedges (optional) | |

1. In a blender or food processor, combine chicken broth, olive oil, garlic, lime juice, Parmesan cheese, almonds, if using, and salt; pulse until a coarse paste forms. Add cilantro and pulse 3 to 4 times, until leaves are broken up but paste is still chunky.
2. Place chicken in a medium bowl. Pour in cilantro mixture and stir until combined.
3. In a medium skillet, heat chicken-and-cilantro mixture over medium heat, stirring occasionally, for about 3 to 4 minutes. Remove from heat, cover and set aside. In a small, dry nonstick skillet over medium heat, heat tortillas for about 30 seconds on each side, until warmed through. (Or, using tongs, char the tortillas directly over a gas stove flame for a few seconds on each side.) Spoon chicken onto tortillas, then add queso fresco and cilantro, if using. Serve with lime wedges to squeeze over tacos, if desired.

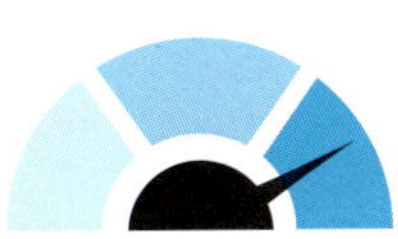


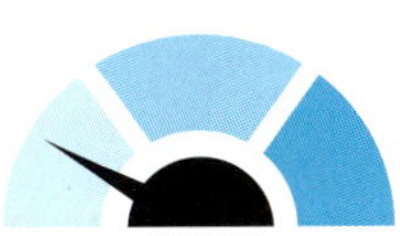


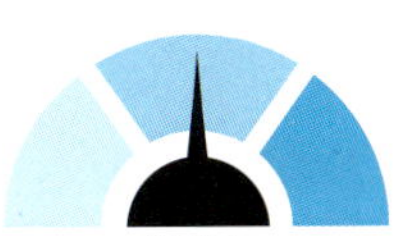


**NUTRIENTS PER SERVING**

| | | | | | |
|---|---|---|---|---|---|
| Calories | 330 kcal | Sodium | 860 mg | Vitamin D | 0 mcg |
| Fat | 14 g | Carbohydrate | 24 g | Calcium | 128 mg |
| Saturated fat | 3.5 g | Fiber | 0 g | Iron | 0 mg |
| Cholesterol | 70 mg | Protein | 25 g | Potassium | 235 mg |

# Chicken Piccata and Peas

▸ LOW CARBOHYDRATE

### MAKES 4 SERVINGS

This is a classic that can be paired with a side salad or a colorful vegetable medley. Choosing leaner proteins, like chicken, is one of the main principles of the Mediterranean diet, which has been linked to better health outcomes for people living with Parkinson's disease.

### TIPS

This recipe is easy to double for a larger crowd.

If you can't find chicken cutlets, make your own by simply cutting boneless skinless chicken breasts in half horizontally to make a thin, even cutlet.

| | | |
|---|---|---|
| 1 lb | thin chicken cutlets or chicken breast slices | 500 g |
| ¼ tsp | salt | 1 mL |
| Pinch | ground black pepper | Pinch |
| ¼ cup | all-purpose flour | 60 mL |
| 3 tbsp | butter, divided | 45 mL |
| 2 tbsp | canola oil | 30 mL |
| 1 cup | ready-to-use chicken broth | 250 mL |
| 1 cup | frozen or fresh peas | 250 mL |
| ½ tsp | grated lemon zest | 2 mL |
| 1 tbsp | freshly squeezed lemon juice | 15 mL |
| 2 tbsp | chopped fresh flat-leaf (Italian) parsley | 30 mL |

1. Sprinkle chicken with salt and pepper. Dredge cutlets in flour to coat and shake off any excess.
2. In large nonstick skillet, melt 2 tbsp (30 mL) of the butter and the oil over medium-high heat and cook cutlets, in batches if necessary, for about 8 minutes or until golden, turning once. Transfer to platter and keep warm.
3. Add broth and peas to skillet and bring to boil. Boil for about 3 minutes or until reduced by half, scraping up brown bits. Add lemon zest and juice, parsley and remaining butter and stir until butter is melted. Return chicken to pan to heat through and simmer for about 2 minutes or until chicken is no longer pink inside.

PROTEIN

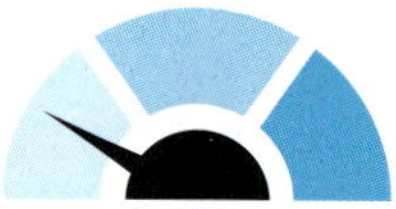
FIBER

SKILL

### NUTRIENTS PER SERVING

| | | | | | |
|---|---|---|---|---|---|
| Calories | 350 kcal | Sodium | 560 mg | Vitamin D | 0 mcg |
| Fat | 19 g | Carbohydrate | 12 g | Calcium | 25 mg |
| Saturated fat | 7 g | Fiber | 2 g | Iron | 1 mg |
| Cholesterol | 115 mg | Protein | 31 g | Potassium | 521 mg |

# Whole Wheat Pasta and Tuna Salad

- LOW CARBOHYDRATE
- MEDITERRANEAN DIET
- MIND DIET

**MAKES 8 SERVINGS**

This is a great way to incorporate fatty fish, which is full of omega-3 fatty acids needed for brain health. Serve some cut-up fresh fruit with low-fat flavored yogurt for dessert.

### TIPS

To prevent the cooked pasta from sticking together, have all the other salad ingredients ready to add as soon as it's drained.

Use canned salmon instead of tuna and add 2 tsp (10 mL) chopped fresh dill.

| | | |
|---|---|---|
| 8 oz | whole wheat fusilli pasta | 250 g |
| 2 | cans (each 6 oz/170 g) water-packed flaked tuna, drained | 2 |
| 3/4 cup | finely chopped red, green or yellow bell pepper (or a combination) | 175 mL |
| 3/4 cup | finely chopped red onion | 175 mL |
| 3/4 cup | coarsely chopped arugula | 175 mL |
| 1/2 cup | cooked green peas | 125 mL |
| 1 cup | low-fat plain yogurt | 250 mL |
| 1/4 cup | light mayonnaise | 60 mL |
| 1 1/2 tsp | Dijon mustard | 7 mL |
| 1 tsp | tarragon vinegar | 5 mL |
| 1/2 tsp | ground black pepper | 2 mL |
| 1/4 tsp | salt | 1 mL |

1. In a large saucepan of boiling salted water, cook pasta according to package directions. Drain and transfer to a large bowl.
2. Add tuna, bell pepper, onion, arugula and peas to pasta and stir to combine. Let cool slightly.
3. In a small bowl, whisk together yogurt, mayonnaise, mustard, vinegar, pepper and salt. Add to pasta mixture and stir well to coat noodles. Cover and refrigerate for at least 4 hours or for up to 8 hours before serving.

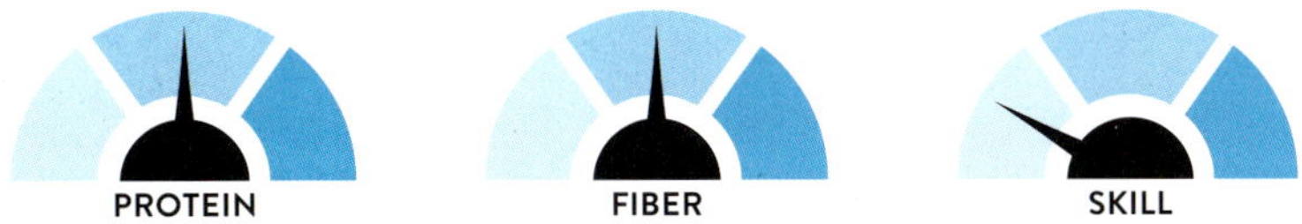


**NUTRIENTS PER SERVING**

| | | | | | |
|---|---|---|---|---|---|
| Calories | 210 kcal | Sodium | 280 mg | Vitamin D | 1 mcg |
| Fat | 5 g | Carbohydrate | 29 g | Calcium | 84 mg |
| Saturated fat | 1 g | Fiber | 4 g | Iron | 2 mg |
| Cholesterol | 20 mg | Protein | 15 g | Potassium | 365 mg |

# Garlic Cilantro Shrimp Tacos

▸ LOW CARBOHYDRATE

**MAKES 4 SERVINGS**

**SERVING SIZE: 2 TACOS**

Some people with tremor might find it difficult to eat a taco. If this is the case, try serving this recipe over a bed of rice with some extra veggies.

**To be gluten-free, be sure to use corn tortillas.*

### TIPS

"Street taco" size tortillas are about 5 inches (12.5 cm), and they are available in flour or corn.

Substitute canned diced tomatoes for the fresh, if needed.

| | | |
|---|---|---|
| 1 lb | large peeled and deveined black tiger shrimp (31/40 count) | 500 g |
| 2 tbsp | canola oil | 30 mL |
| 2 tbsp | chopped fresh cilantro | 30 mL |
| 2 | cloves garlic, minced | 2 |
| 2 tsp | smoked paprika | 10 mL |
| 1 cup | diced tomato | 250 mL |
| 1/4 tsp | salt | 1 mL |
| 1/2 tsp | grated lime zest | 2 mL |
| 1 tbsp | freshly squeezed lime juice | 15 mL |
| 8 | 5 inch (12.5 cm) corn or flour tortillas | 8 |
| 1/2 cup | shredded jalapeño Havarti or Gouda cheese | 125 mL |
| | Lime wedges (optional) | |

1. Remove tails from shrimp. In a large bowl, toss shrimp with oil, cilantro, garlic and paprika. Let stand for 10 minutes.
2. Meanwhile, heat a large nonstick skillet over medium-high heat; add tomato and salt. Cook, stirring, for about 2 minutes or until tomatoes start to soften. Add shrimp mixture and stir to combine. Cook for about 5 minutes or until shrimp are pink and firm. Stir in lime zest and juice and remove from heat.
3. Divide mixture among tortillas and sprinkle each with cheese to serve. Serve with lime wedges, if desired.

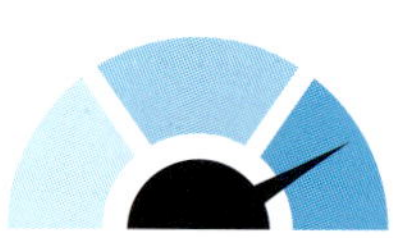
PROTEIN

FIBER

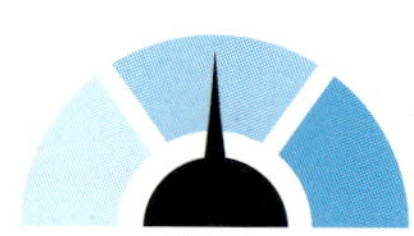
SKILL

**NUTRIENTS PER SERVING**

| | | | | | |
|---|---|---|---|---|---|
| Calories | 360 kcal | Sodium | 420 mg | Vitamin D | 0 mcg |
| Fat | 15 g | Carbohydrate | 28 g | Calcium | 161 mg |
| Saturated fat | 3 g | Fiber | 1 g | Iron | 2 mg |
| Cholesterol | 180 mg | Protein | 29 g | Potassium | 146 mg |

# Maple Soy Salmon

- DYSPHAGIA-FRIENDLY
- HIGH CALORIE
- MEDITERRANEAN DIET

**MAKES 2 SERVINGS**

**SERVING SIZE: 6 OZ (175 G)**

Omega-3 fatty acids from the salmon could help reduce inflammation as part of a well-balanced diet. This recipe is higher in sodium for those that need help managing orthostatic hypotension.

### TIP

Salmon provides omega-3 fats, which help support heart, brain and eye health at all stages of life. Aim for eating at least 7 oz (210 g) of fatty fish per week.

- **Baking sheet, brushed with 1 tsp (5 mL) olive oil**

| | | |
|---|---|---|
| **1 tbsp** | **reduced-sodium soy sauce** | **15 mL** |
| **1 tsp** | **pure maple syrup** | **5 mL** |
| **2 tsp** | **olive oil** | **10 mL** |
| **1⁄8 tsp** | **ground black pepper** | **0.5 mL** |
| **12 oz** | **salmon fillet, with the skin on** | **375 g** |

1. In a large bowl, add the soy sauce, maple syrup, oil and pepper and whisk until combined. Add the salmon and turn to evenly coat. Cover the bowl and place in the refrigerator for at least 20 minutes and up to 4 hours.
2. Preheat the oven to 350°F (180°C).
3. Place the salmon, skin side down, onto the prepared baking sheet. Discard the leftover marinade. Bake until the fish is opaque and flaky, 15 minutes.

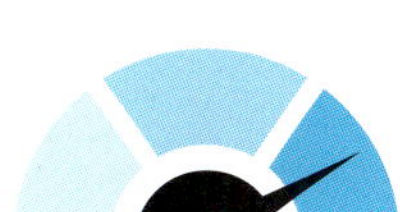
PROTEIN

FIBER

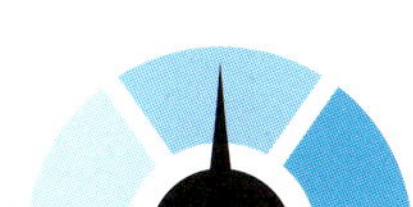
SKILL

**NUTRIENTS PER SERVING**

| | | | | | |
|---|---|---|---|---|---|
| Calories | 430 kcal | Sodium | 1,330 mg | Vitamin D | 0 mcg |
| Fat | 19 g | Carbohydrate | 43 g | Calcium | 32 mg |
| Saturated fat | 3.5 g | Fiber | 0 g | Iron | 3 mg |
| Cholesterol | 35 mg | Protein | 19 g | Potassium | 301 mg |

# Roasted Mushroom Penne

MEDITERRANEAN DIET

**MAKES 6 SERVINGS**

This recipe has a fun blend of many mushroom varieties, providing a source of vitamin D, which is essential for bone health.

## TIPS

If the button mushrooms are large, cut them in half or even into quarters before roasting.

To trim the portobello mushrooms, cut off the bottom ½ inch (1 cm) of the stem.

The quantity of garlic depends on the size of the cloves. If large, use the smaller number. If small, more may be required.

- Baking sheet, lined with parchment paper
- Preheat oven to 450°F (230°C)

| | | |
|---|---|---|
| 4 cups | whole button mushrooms (see Tips, left) | 1 L |
| 4 cups | sliced portobello mushrooms (see Tips, left) | 1 L |
| 2 cups | thickly sliced shiitake mushroom caps | 500 mL |
| 2 cups | thickly sliced oyster mushrooms | 500 mL |
| 6 tbsp | grapeseed oil, divided | 90 mL |
| 3 tbsp | chopped fresh thyme leaves | 45 mL |
| 1½ tsp | fine sea salt, divided | 7 mL |
| 1 | package (16 oz/500 g) gluten-free penne | 1 |
| ½ cup | chopped onion | 125 mL |
| 3 to 4 | cloves garlic, minced (see Tips, left) | 3 to 4 |

1. In a large bowl, toss together button, portobello, shiitake and oyster mushrooms, 3 tbsp (45 mL) oil, thyme and 1 tsp (5 mL) salt. Transfer to prepared baking sheet. Bake in preheated oven until mushrooms are soft and lightly browned, about 30 minutes. Transfer mushrooms and their liquid to a large bowl. Set aside.

2. In a large covered saucepan, bring water to a rapid boil (see Tips, opposite). Add remaining ½ tsp (2 mL) salt and penne and cook, uncovered, until pasta is al dente. Scoop out ½ cup (125 mL) cooking water and set aside (see Tips, opposite). Drain.

PROTEIN

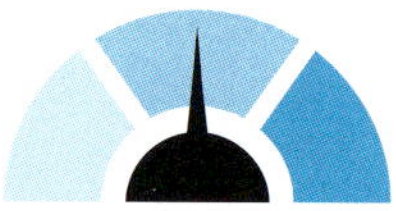
FIBER

SKILL

**NUTRIENTS PER SERVING**

| | | | | | |
|---|---|---|---|---|---|
| Calories | 340 kcal | Sodium | 610 mg | Vitamin D | 1 mcg |
| Fat | 15 g | Carbohydrate | 47 g | Calcium | 17 mg |
| Saturated fat | 2 g | Fiber | 5 g | Iron | 2 mg |
| Cholesterol | 0 mg | Protein | 8 g | Potassium | 584 mg |

## TIPS

Gluten-free pasta needs to be cooked in a lot of rapidly boiling water so it does not stick together. Make sure you use a large saucepan with at least 4 to 5 times more water than pasta.

The residual starch in pasta cooking water helps to thicken and add body to the sauce. Chefs usually scoop out a quantity before draining pasta. Then they add 1/4 to 1/2 cup (60 to 125 mL) to the sauce, depending upon the desired result.

3. Meanwhile, in a large skillet over medium heat, heat remaining 3 tbsp (45 mL) oil. Add onion and cook, stirring frequently, until translucent, about 6 minutes. Add garlic and cook until fragrant, about 2 minutes. Stir in roasted mushrooms and liquid.

4. Add reserved penne and pasta water to the skillet. Using a wooden spoon, stir to coat evenly. Serve immediately.

CHAPTER 13

# DINNER

# Florentine Pizza

**MAKES 4 SERVINGS**

**SERVING SIZE: 1½ NAAN**

This is a simpler twist on a homemade pizza. Using naan saves time compared to making a pizza from scratch. Pizza makes for a balanced dinner too! Just add nutrients by piling your favorite vegetables on top!

## TIPS

Substitute vegan shredded cheese for the mozzarella.

You can substitute 4 regular-size naan for the 6 mini naan breads. (Mini naan are larger than naan dippers.)

Top it with a fried egg for some vegetarian protein.

- Preheat oven to 400°F (200°C)

| | | |
|---|---|---|
| 1 tbsp | canola oil | 15 mL |
| 1 | small onion, diced | 1 |
| 2 | cloves garlic, minced | 2 |
| 1 | small red bell pepper, chopped | 1 |
| 2 tsp | dried oregano | 10 mL |
| 1 | package (11 oz/312 g) fresh baby spinach | 1 |
| ¼ tsp | salt | 1 mL |
| ¼ tsp | ground black pepper | 1 mL |
| 6 | mini naan breads (see Tips, left) | 6 |
| ½ cup | pizza or pasta sauce | 125 mL |
| 1 cup | shredded mozzarella cheese | 250 mL |

1. In a large nonstick skillet, heat oil over medium heat. Cook onion, garlic, red pepper and oregano, stirring for about 5 minutes or until softened. Add spinach and cook, stirring for about 3 minutes or until spinach is wilted. Drain any water if necessary. Stir in salt and pepper.
2. Place naan on large baking sheet and spread each with pizza sauce. Spread spinach mixture over top of each bread. Sprinkle with cheese. Bake for about 8 minutes or until cheese is melted and naan are golden.

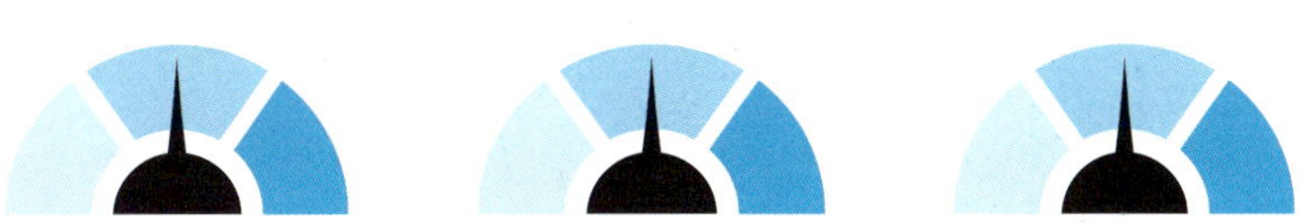


**NUTRIENTS PER SERVING**

| | | | | | |
|---|---|---|---|---|---|
| Calories | 316 kcal | Sodium | 1,060 mg | Vitamin D | 0 mcg |
| Fat | 10 g | Carbohydrate | 43 g | Calcium | 450 mg |
| Saturated fat | 2 g | Fiber | 4 g | Iron | 4 mg |
| Cholesterol | 13 mg | Protein | 18 g | Potassium | 724 mg |

# Black Bean Burgers

- DYSPHAGIA-FRIENDLY
- LOW CARBOHYDRATE
- MEDITERRANEAN DIET
- MIND DIET

**MAKES 8 BURGERS**

**SERVING SIZE: 1 BURGER**

This plant-based burger could be easier on those with medication–dietary protein interactions. Pair this burger with sweet potato fries or a side salad for a balanced meal.

### TIP

**To soak the beans:** Place them in a bowl with 8 cups (2 L) water. Cover and set aside for at least 6 hours or overnight (if overnight, refrigerate). Drain, discarding water.

- Food processor
- Baking sheet, lined with parchment paper

| | | |
|---|---|---|
| 9 cups | water, divided | 2.25 L |
| 2 cups | black beans, soaked (see Tips, left) | 500 mL |
| ½ cup | millet, rinsed and drained | 125 mL |
| 1 tbsp | grapeseed oil | 15 mL |
| 1 | medium onion, thinly sliced | 1 |
| 1 tsp | chili powder | 5 mL |
| ½ tsp | ground cumin | 2 mL |
| ¼ cup | ketchup | 60 mL |
| 3 tbsp | wheat-free tamari | 45 mL |
| ¼ cup | raw sunflower seeds | 60 mL |
| ½ cup | brown rice flour | 125 mL |
| ¼ cup | ground raw flax seeds | 60 mL |

1. In a large saucepan, combine 6 cups (1.5 L) water and beans and bring to a boil. Reduce heat and simmer until beans are tender, about 1 hour. Drain, discarding water. Transfer to a large bowl and set aside.
2. Meanwhile, in another saucepan, combine millet and 3 cups (750 mL) water and bring to a boil. Reduce heat and simmer, until millet is tender and almost all of the liquid has been absorbed about 15 minutes. Cover and set aside.

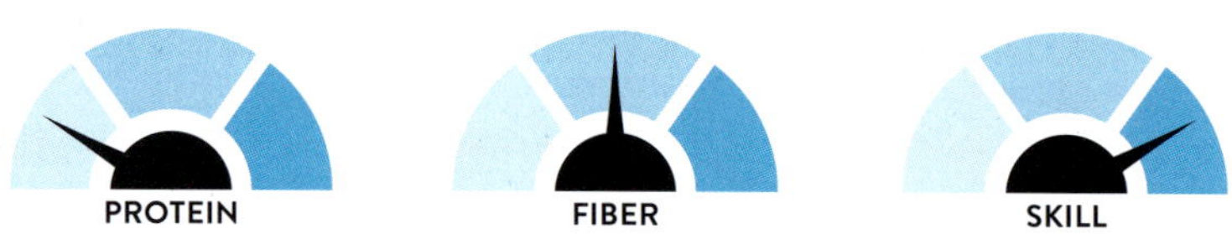


**NUTRIENTS PER SERVING**

| | | | | | |
|---|---|---|---|---|---|
| Calories | 190 kcal | Sodium | 560 mg | Vitamin D | 0 mcg |
| Fat | 7 g | Carbohydrate | 26 g | Calcium | 26 mg |
| Saturated fat | 1 g | Fiber | 6 g | Iron | 2 mg |
| Cholesterol | 0 mg | Protein | 6 g | Potassium | 243 mg |

**TIP**

You can use either brown or golden flax seeds in this recipe. To grind the flax for this recipe, process 3 tbsp (45 mL) whole raw flax seeds to a powder in either a clean spice grinder or a blender.

3. In a skillet over medium heat, heat oil. Sauté onion until lightly golden, 3 to 4 minutes. Stir in chili powder and cumin and cook for 1 to 2 minutes, until fragrant. Stir in ketchup and tamari and simmer for 2 to 3 minutes. Remove from heat and set aside to cool slightly. Add to reserved beans, along with millet and sunflower seeds. Toss to combine.
4. Preheat oven to 400°F (200°C).
5. Transfer bean mixture to food processor fitted with the metal blade (reserve bowl) and process until smooth, stopping the motor to scrape down sides of work bowl as necessary. Return to bowl. Add rice flour and ground flax seeds and stir until well incorporated.
6. Dip a ½-cup (125 mL) ladle or measuring cup in water, then scoop 8 equal portions of bean mixture onto prepared baking sheet, rewetting ladle as necessary. Using your hands, form burgers to desired shape.
7. Bake in preheated oven for 15 to 20 minutes or until lightly golden on the bottom and firm in the middle. Serve immediately or transfer to an airtight container and refrigerate for up to 1 week. To reheat, place on a rimmed baking sheet lined with parchment paper, and warm in oven preheated to 350°F (180°C) until heated through, about 10 minutes.

# Tofu-Pepper Teriyaki Kebabs

- KETOGENIC DIET
- LOW CARBOHYDRATE
- MEDITERRANEAN DIET
- MIND DIET

**MAKES 4 SERVINGS**

**SERVING SIZE: 2 SKEWERS**

This is a simple plant-based protein option that can be paired with brown or wild rice for an extra boost of carbohydrates. Red bell pepper adds color and flavor, but you can add even more fruits and vegetables to your liking! Some ideas include zucchini, pineapple and/or red onion.

- 8 wooden skewers
- Grill pan or grill

| | | |
|---|---|---|
| 8 oz | extra-firm tofu, drained | 250 g |
| ¼ cup | teriyaki sauce | 60 mL |
| 2 | red bell peppers, cut into 2- by 1-inch (5 by 2.5 cm) strips | 2 |
| 1 tbsp | extra-virgin olive oil | 15 mL |

1. Cut the tofu into 1-inch (2.5 cm) cubes and place in a large bowl. Add the teriyaki sauce and toss to evenly coat. Cover the bowl and place in the refrigerator for at least 1 hour and up to 4 hours.
2. Soak wooden skewers in water for 10 minutes before threading.
3. Preheat a grill pan or grill to medium-high heat. Brush the oil onto the grill pan or grates of the grill.
4. Thread each skewer with about 3 pieces each of tofu and 3 pieces of pepper, alternating between the two.
5. Grill until the tofu and pepper are slightly browned, 7 to 8 minutes, turning halfway through.
6. Serve warm.

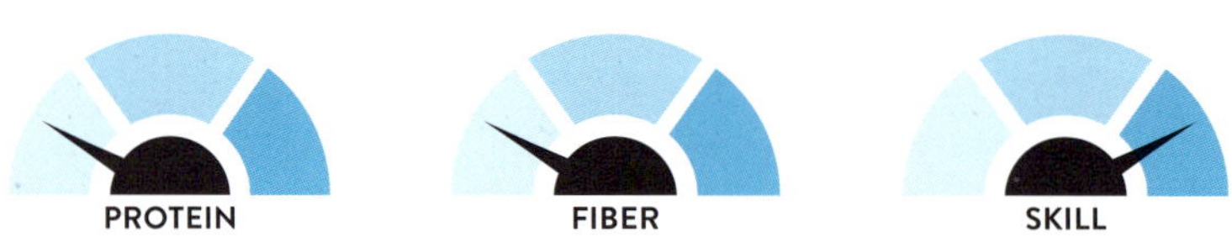


**NUTRIENTS PER SERVING**

| | | | | | |
|---|---|---|---|---|---|
| Calories | 130 kcal | Sodium | 400 mg | Vitamin D | 0 mcg |
| Fat | 7 g | Carbohydrate | 8 g | Calcium | 104 mg |
| Saturated fat | 1 g | Fiber | 1 g | Iron | 1 mg |
| Cholesterol | 0 mg | Protein | 8 g | Potassium | 126 mg |

# Polenta and Cheese–Stuffed Peppers

**MAKES 6 SERVINGS**

**SERVING SIZE: 1 STUFFED PEPPER HALF**

Bell peppers are a great vessel for balanced meals! This vegetarian dinner has moderate amounts of protein and fiber to support overall health.

### TIP

To make it ahead, cover the casserole dish before baking and refrigerate for up to 1 day. Add about 10 minutes to the oven time when reheating.

- Preheat oven to 400°F (200°C)

| | | |
|---|---|---|
| 2 tbsp | canola oil | 30 mL |
| 1 | onion, diced | 1 |
| 1 | zucchini, diced | 1 |
| 4 | cloves garlic, minced | 4 |
| Pinch | hot pepper flakes | Pinch |
| 2 cups | ready-to-use vegetable broth | 500 mL |
| ½ cup | cornmeal | 125 mL |
| ¼ cup | chopped fresh parsley | 60 mL |
| 1½ cups | shredded mozzarella-Cheddar cheese blend, divided | 375 mL |
| 1½ cups | tomato basil pasta sauce | 375 mL |
| 3 | red bell peppers, halved, seeds and membranes removed | 3 |

1. In a large skillet, heat oil over medium heat. Cook onion, zucchini, garlic and hot pepper flakes for 5 minutes or until softened. Pour in broth and bring to a boil. Whisk in cornmeal and cook on low heat, stirring, for about 15 minutes or until very thick. Stir in parsley; remove from heat. Stir in 1 cup (250 mL) of the cheese.

2. Pour pasta sauce into bottom of 11- by 7-inch (28 by 18 cm) casserole dish. Spoon polenta filling into pepper halves and place into casserole dish. Cover with foil and bake for about 35 minutes or until peppers are tender. Uncover and sprinkle with remaining cheese and bake for 10 minutes or until cheese is golden and bubbly.

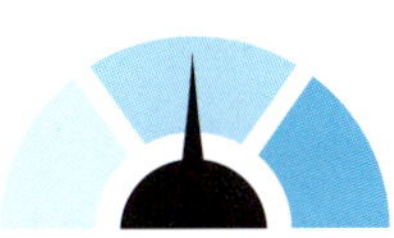
PROTEIN

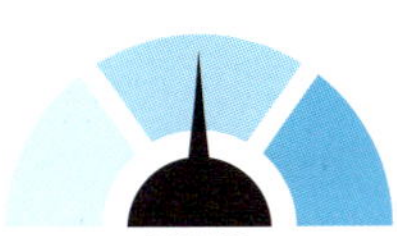
FIBER

SKILL

**NUTRIENTS PER SERVING**

| | | | | | |
|---|---|---|---|---|---|
| Calories | 273 kcal | Sodium | 623 mg | Vitamin D | 0 mcg |
| Fat | 12 g | Carbohydrate | 32 g | Calcium | 301 mg |
| Saturated fat | 4 g | Fiber | 5 g | Iron | 1 mg |
| Cholesterol | 16 mg | Protein | 12 g | Potassium | 847 mg |

# Whole Wheat Mac and Cheese

▸ DYSPHAGIA-FRIENDLY

**MAKES 8 SERVINGS**

This vegetarian-friendly dinner is full of protein and calcium to support muscle and bone health. Use olive oil, low-fat cheese and whole wheat pasta to adhere closer to a Mediterranean diet.

### TIP

To make fresh bread crumbs, slice bread, cut off the crusts, break into chunks and process in a food processor fitted with a metal blade until desired consistency is reached.

- Preheat oven to 375°F (190°C)
- 8-cup (2 L) baking dish, greased

| | | |
|---|---|---|
| 2 cups | whole wheat penne | 500 mL |
| 1 tbsp | extra-virgin olive oil | 15 mL |
| 2 cups | shredded sharp (old) Cheddar cheese, divided | 500 mL |
| ½ cup | freshly grated Parmesan cheese, divided | 125 mL |
| 1 cup | fresh whole wheat bread crumbs (see Tip, left) | 250 mL |
| ¼ cup | butter, divided | 60 mL |
| ¼ cup | whole wheat or all-purpose flour | 60 mL |
| 1½ tsp | chipotle chile powder (see Tip, opposite) | 7 mL |
| 1 tsp | dried oregano, crumbled | 5 mL |
| 3 cups | warm milk | 750 mL |
| 1 tbsp | Dijon mustard | 15 mL |
| 1 cup | shredded reduced-fat Swiss or Gruyère cheese | 250 mL |
| | Salt and ground black pepper | |
| 3 | tomatoes, thinly sliced, optional | 3 |

1. In a saucepan of boiling salted water, cook penne until tender to the bite, about 12 minutes. Drain and rinse well under cold running water. Transfer to a bowl and toss with olive oil.
2. In another bowl, mix together ¼ cup (60 mL) of the Cheddar, 2 tbsp (30 mL) of the Parmesan and bread crumbs. Set aside.

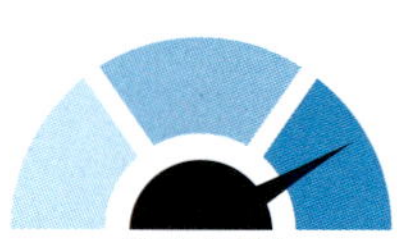
PROTEIN

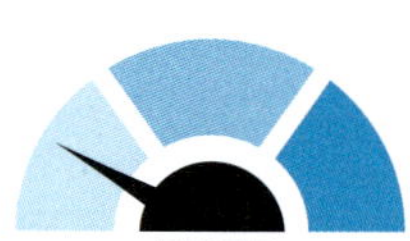
FIBER

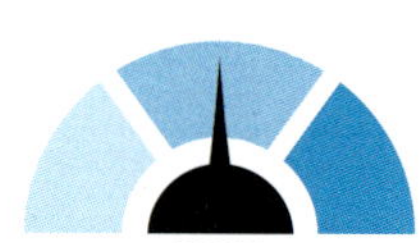
SKILL

**NUTRIENTS PER SERVING**

| | | | | | |
|---|---|---|---|---|---|
| Calories | 356 kcal | Sodium | 741 mg | Vitamin D | 1 mcg |
| Fat | 19 g | Carbohydrate | 27 g | Calcium | 515 mg |
| Saturated fat | 8 g | Fiber | 3 g | Iron | 2 mg |
| Cholesterol | 42 mg | Protein | 20 g | Potassium | 328 mg |

### TIP

Chipotle chile powder is available in well-stocked supermarkets and specialty stores. Or you can make your own by grinding a dried chipotle chile pepper in a spice grinder. For a milder result, use ancho chile, New Mexico chile or a traditional blended chili powder.

3. In a large saucepan, melt 3 tbsp (45 mL) of the butter over medium heat. Add flour and cook, stirring, until foamy. Continue cooking and stirring, without browning, for 1 minute. Stir in chipotle chile powder and oregano. Gradually add warm milk, whisking until blended. Continue to cook, stirring, until mixture comes to a boil and thickens, about 7 minutes. Whisk in mustard.
4. Reduce heat to low. Add Swiss cheese and remaining Cheddar and Parmesan cheeses and cook, stirring, until melted and smooth. Season to taste with salt and pepper. Remove from heat and stir in reserved pasta.
5. Transfer pasta mixture to prepared dish, spreading evenly. Arrange tomatoes, if using, evenly over top, in layers, as necessary. Sprinkle bread crumb mixture evenly over top. Melt remaining 1 tbsp (15 mL) of butter and drizzle over top. Bake in preheated oven until hot and bubbly, about 25 minutes. Preheat broiler and broil until crumbs are crisp and browned, about 2 minutes.

# Eggplant Parm

**MAKES 4 SERVINGS**

The perfect vegan or vegetarian meal for someone following a plant-based diet! This recipe can be made with a low-fat cheese for those that do not follow a vegan diet.

- **Preheat the oven to 400°F (200°C)**
- **Large rimmed baking sheet, lined with parchment paper**

| | | |
|---|---|---|
| **½ cup** | **unsweetened nondairy milk** | **125 mL** |
| **1¼ cups** | **panko bread crumbs** | **310 mL** |
| **⅓ cup** | **all-purpose flour** | **75 mL** |
| **¼ cup** | **vegan Parmesan cheese or nutritional yeast** | **60 mL** |
| **¼ tsp** | **salt** | **1 mL** |
| **1** | **large eggplant (approx. 1 lb/500 g), sliced into 12 (½ inch/1 cm) rounds** | **1** |
| | **Cooking spray (optional)** | |
| **1½ cups** | **store-bought marinara sauce** | **375 mL** |
| **2 cups** | **vegan mozzarella cheese shreds** | **500 mL** |

1. Pour the nondairy milk into a large bowl. Set aside.
2. In another large bowl, whisk together the panko, flour, vegan Parmesan and salt.
3. Submerge a slice of eggplant in the nondairy milk, then dip into the panko mixture, turning until all sides are coated. Gently shake off the excess crumbs. Place on the prepared baking sheet. Repeat with the remaining slices, making a single layer. Discard excess nondairy milk and panko mixture.

PROTEIN

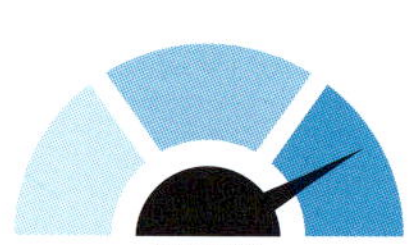
FIBER

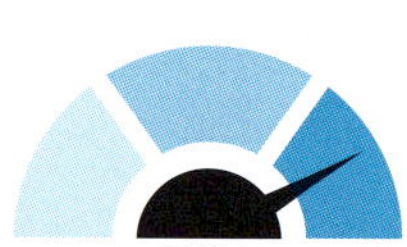
SKILL

**NUTRIENTS PER SERVING**

| | | | | | |
|---|---|---|---|---|---|
| Calories | 409 kcal | Sodium | 1,049 mg | Vitamin D | 0 mcg |
| Fat | 15 g | Carbohydrate | 57 g | Calcium | 67 mg |
| Saturated fat | 13 g | Fiber | 8 g | Iron | 2 mg |
| Cholesterol | 0 mg | Protein | 10 g | Potassium | 407 mg |

### TIP

If you prefer the eggplant coating to stay crispy, skip adding the marinara sauce in Step 5. Sprinkle the vegan cheese directly over the eggplant and bake as directed. Meanwhile, heat the marinara sauce separately in a small saucepan over medium-low heat for about 5 minutes, stirring frequently, until warm. Spoon over the eggplant slices just before serving.

4. Spray the eggplant slices with cooking spray (if using). Bake in the preheated oven for 15 minutes or until golden brown on the bottom, then flip and bake for 10 minutes more, until golden brown on the other side.

5. Spoon the marinara sauce evenly over the slices, then sprinkle with the vegan mozzarella cheese. Bake for 10 minutes or until cheese is melted. Remove from the oven and let cool slightly before serving.

# Quick and Easy Lentil Tacos

- MEDITERRANEAN DIET
- MIND DIET

**MAKES 4 SERVINGS**

**SERVING SIZE: 1 TACO**

This one-pan meal is a great option for people that have difficulty standing in the kitchen for long periods of time. Pro tip: Use a vegetable chopper to save time and energy preparing the vegetables in this recipe.

### TIPS

You can use 1 can (19 oz/540 mL) lentils, drained and rinsed, instead of cooked lentils.

To make a taco salad, spoon the lentil filling on top of a bed of lettuce and tomato, then sprinkle with cheese and garnish with baked tortilla chips.

| | | |
|---|---|---|
| 1½ cups | cooked green lentils (see Tips, left) | 375 mL |
| 2 tbsp | minced red onion | 30 mL |
| 2 tbsp | minced red bell pepper | 30 mL |
| ¼ cup | salsa | 60 mL |
| 4 | corn taco shells | 4 |
| ¾ cup | finely shredded romaine or iceberg lettuce | 175 mL |
| ¾ cup | diced plum (Roma) tomatoes | 175 mL |
| ½ cup | shredded Cheddar or light Cheddar cheese | 125 mL |
| ½ cup | light sour cream (optional) | 125 mL |
| 1 | avocado, cubed (optional) | 1 |
| ½ cup | sliced black olives (optional) | 125 mL |

1. In a medium saucepan over medium heat, combine lentils, onion, red pepper and salsa; cook, stirring often, for 3 to 4 minutes or until bubbling and hot.
2. Fill each taco shell with one-quarter of the lentil mixture, lettuce, tomato and cheese. If desired, top with sour cream, avocado and olives.

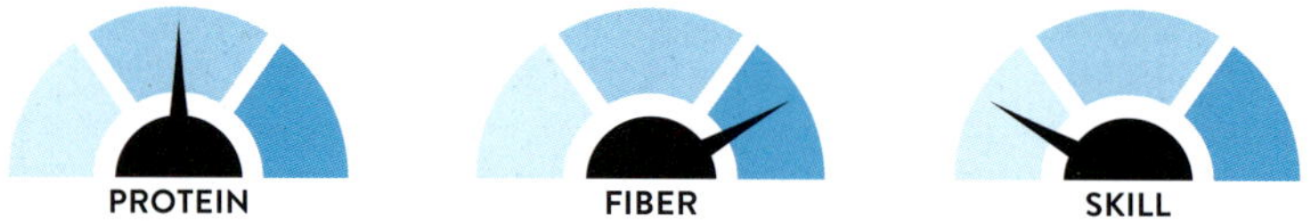


**NUTRIENTS PER SERVING**

| | | | | | |
|---|---|---|---|---|---|
| Calories | 243 kcal | Sodium | 386 mg | Vitamin D | 0 mcg |
| Fat | 7 g | Carbohydrate | 33 g | Calcium | 158 mg |
| Saturated fat | 3 g | Fiber | 9 g | Iron | 3 mg |
| Cholesterol | 8 mg | Protein | 13 g | Potassium | 483 mg |

# Black Bean Enchilada Casserole

- DYSPHAGIA-FRIENDLY
- HIGH CALORIE
- MEDITERRANEAN DIET

**MAKES 8 SERVINGS**

This plant-based casserole is ideal for those looking for an effortless weeknight dinner. It's full of protein and fiber to support muscle and gastrointestinal health. Use a Mediterranean-diet approach by choosing olive oil and opting for low-fat cheese.

## TIPS

For non-vegetarians, substitute 1 lb (500 g) cooked lean ground beef or 4 boneless skinless chicken breasts, cooked and shredded, for the black beans.

You can replace the corn tortillas with flour tortillas.

- Preheat oven to 250°F (120°C)
- 13- by 9-inch (33 by 23 cm) glass baking dish, greased

| | | |
|---|---|---|
| 2 tbsp | olive oil or butter | 30 mL |
| 1 | onion, finely chopped | 1 |
| 2 | cans (each 14 to 19 oz/398 to 540 mL) black beans, drained and rinsed | 2 |
| 1 | can (4½ oz/127 mL) chopped mild green chiles | 1 |
| 1 | can (10 oz/284 mL) enchilada sauce | 1 |
| 1 cup | sour cream | 250 mL |
| 30 | 6- or 7-inch (15 or 18 cm) corn tortillas | 30 |
| 3 cups | shredded Cheddar cheese, divided | 750 mL |

1. In a large nonstick skillet, heat oil over medium-high heat. Sauté onion for 5 to 7 minutes or until tender. Stir in beans, chiles, enchilada sauce and sour cream; cook until heated through.
2. Tear tortillas into bite-size pieces. Layer half the tortilla pieces in prepared baking dish. Spoon in half the bean mixture and layer with half the cheese. Repeat layers, ending with cheese.
3. Bake in preheated oven for 40 to 45 minutes or until bubbling.

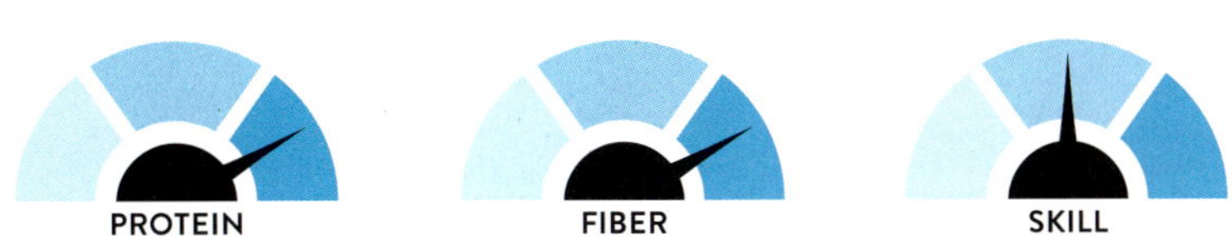


**NUTRIENTS PER SERVING**

| | | | | | |
|---|---|---|---|---|---|
| Calories | 630 kcal | Sodium | 870 mg | Vitamin D | 0 mcg |
| Fat | 25 g | Carbohydrate | 77 g | Calcium | 537 mg |
| Saturated fat | 6 g | Fiber | 10 g | Iron | 4 mg |
| Cholesterol | 25 mg | Protein | 27 g | Potassium | 635 mg |

# Pinto Bean Tortilla Soup

- MEDITERRANEAN DIET
- MIND DIET

**MAKES 8 SERVINGS**

This classic bean soup combines a variety of plant proteins, vegetables and spices for a flavorful, nutrient-dense meal. With a moderate amount of protein and fiber, this soup supports muscle and gut health.

### TIP

The tomatoes and onions can be broiled up to 1 day in advance. Let cool, cover and refrigerate until ready to use.

- Rimmed baking sheet
- Food processor or blender

| | | |
|---|---|---|
| 1½ cups | dried pinto beans | 375 mL |
| 1 | large onion, cut into 6 wedges | 1 |
| 5 | plum (Roma) tomatoes, quartered | 5 |
| 4 tsp | canola oil, divided | 20 mL |
| 4 | 5-inch (12.5 cm) corn tortillas | 4 |
| 2 | cloves garlic, minced | 2 |
| 1 | jalapeño pepper, seeded and finely minced | 1 |
| 2 tsp | ground cumin | 10 mL |
| 1 tsp | ground coriander | 5 mL |
| 4 cups | reduced-sodium chicken broth | 1 L |
| 1 | bay leaf | 1 |
| 2 tbsp | tomato paste | 30 mL |
| 1 cup | frozen corn kernels | 250 mL |
| Pinch | salt | Pinch |
| ½ | avocado, chopped | ½ |
| ½ cup | shredded Cheddar cheese | 125 mL |

1. Place beans in a large bowl and add enough cold water to cover by at least 3 inches (7.5 cm). Cover and let soak overnight. Drain soaked beans and rinse well under cold water. Discard any shriveled beans or those that did not swell.

PROTEIN

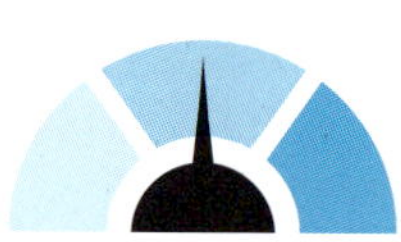
FIBER

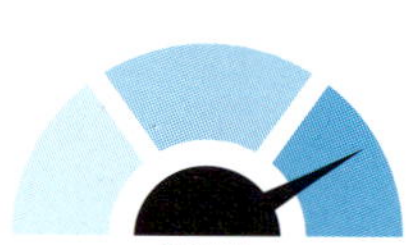
SKILL

**NUTRIENTS PER SERVING**

| | | | | | |
|---|---|---|---|---|---|
| Calories | 200 kcal | Sodium | 150 mg | Vitamin D | 0 mcg |
| Fat | 3 g | Carbohydrate | 33 g | Calcium | 76 mg |
| Saturated fat | 0 g | Fiber | 7 g | Iron | 1 mg |
| Cholesterol | 0 mg | Protein | 10 g | Potassium | 291 mg |

**TIP**

It's impossible to tell the hotness of a jalapeño pepper by looking at it. One way to test for hotness is to place the tip of your finger on a cut piece of jalapeño and touch your finger to your tongue. Be sure to wash your hand afterward, and don't touch your eyes.

2. Place beans in a large saucepan and add enough fresh cold water to cover by 3 inches (7.5 cm). Bring to a boil over high heat. Reduce heat and simmer for 30 to 35 minutes or until beans are tender. Drain and set aside.

3. Meanwhile, preheat broiler. Place onion and tomatoes on a rimmed baking sheet and brush with 1 tsp (5 mL) of the oil. Broil, turning every 5 minutes, for about 15 minutes or until charred. Transfer to food processor and process until smooth. Set aside. Reduce oven temperature to 350°F (180°C). Wipe off the baking sheet and set aside.

4. Cut tortillas into 2- by ¼-inch (5 by 0.5 cm) strips.

5. In a clean large saucepan, heat 2 tsp (10 mL) oil over medium heat. Add half the tortilla strips, garlic and jalapeño; sauté for 3 minutes. Stir in cumin and coriander. Add broth and deglaze the pot, scraping up any brown bits stuck to the bottom. Add bay leaf and bring to a boil. Stir in puréed onion mixture and tomato paste; return to a boil. Reduce heat and simmer, stirring occasionally, for 20 minutes. Stir in corn and cooked pinto beans; simmer for 10 minutes to blend the flavors. Discard bay leaf.

6. Meanwhile, gently toss the remaining tortilla strips with the remaining 1 tsp (5 mL) oil and the salt. Spread on the reserved baking sheet. Bake for about 10 minutes or until crisp.

7. Ladle soup into bowls and garnish with baked tortilla strips, avocado and cheese.

# Tuna Pasta with Capers and Lemon

- KETOGENIC DIET
- LOW CARBOHYDRATE
- MEDITERRANEAN DIET

**MAKES 1 SERVING**

**SERVING SIZE: 16-OZ (500 ML) MUG**

This recipe uses mostly nonperishable ingredients and just requires a microwave for cooking. It's the perfect balanced recipe for someone that has difficulty using a heating element.

### TIP

Add 1⁄4 tsp (1 mL) of your favorite dried herbs or herb blend (dill, basil, oregano, Italian seasoning) with the tuna.

| | | |
|---|---|---|
| 1⁄3 cup | orzo or other small pasta | 75 mL |
| 1⁄8 tsp | salt | 0.5 mL |
| 2⁄3 cup | water | 150 mL |
| 1⁄2 | can (6 oz/170 g) water-packed chunk white tuna, drained and flaked | 1⁄2 |
| 1 tbsp | olive oil | 15 mL |
| 2 tsp | drained capers | 10 mL |
| 1⁄2 tsp | finely grated lemon zest | 2 mL |
| 2 tsp | freshly squeezed lemon juice | 10 mL |
| | Salt and ground black pepper | |
| 1 tbsp | chopped fresh parsley (optional) | 15 mL |

1. In a 16-oz (500 mL) mug, combine orzo, salt and water. Place in the microwave atop a doubled paper towel. Microwave on High for 2 minutes. Stir. Microwave on High for 3 minutes. If the mixture appears dry, add 1 tbsp (15 mL) water to the mug. Microwave for 1½ to 2 minutes or until orzo is tender.
2. Stir in tuna, oil, capers, lemon zest and lemon juice. Microwave on High for 45 to 75 seconds or until heated through. Let stand for 1 minute, then stir. Season to taste with salt and pepper. If desired, stir in parsley.

### CHICKEN PASTA WITH CAPERS AND LEMON

Use half a 5-oz (142 g) can of water-packed chunk chicken, drained and flaked, in place of the tuna.

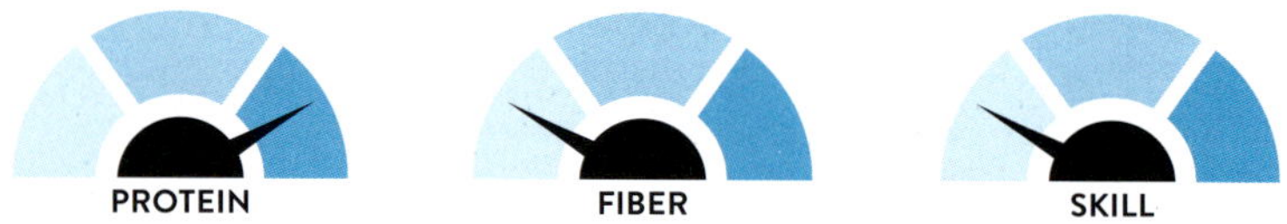


**NUTRIENTS PER SERVING**

| | | | | | |
|---|---|---|---|---|---|
| Calories | 266 kcal | Sodium | 624 mg | Vitamin D | 1 mcg |
| Fat | 15 g | Carbohydrate | 15 g | Calcium | 20 mg |
| Saturated fat | 2 g | Fiber | 1 g | Iron | 2 mg |
| Cholesterol | 31 mg | Protein | 18 g | Potassium | 204 mg |

# Savory Salmon in Foil

- DYSPHAGIA-FRIENDLY
- KETOGENIC DIET
- LOW CARBOHYDRATE
- MEDITERRANEAN DIET
- MIND DIET

**MAKES 6 SERVINGS**

**SERVING SIZE: JUST OVER 5 OZ (150 G)**

Pair with a whole grain, like wild rice, and vegetables for a balanced meal.

- Preheat oven to 400°F (200°C)

| | | |
|---|---|---|
| 2 lbs | salmon fillet, cut into 6 equal pieces | 1 kg |
| 2 | medium lemons | 2 |
| 1 tbsp | olive oil | 15 mL |
| 1 tsp | sea salt | 5 mL |
| 1 tsp | dried rosemary | 5 mL |
| 1 tsp | dried dill | 5 mL |
| 12 to 15 | whole pink peppercorns (optional) | 12 to 15 |
| 1½ tsp | butter | 7 mL |

1. Cut six 12-inch (30 cm) squares of foil. Lay out squares on a flat surface and place one salmon piece in center of each.
2. Cut six ¼-inch (0.5 cm) thick slices crosswise out of center of each lemon. Using ends of the lemons, squeeze equal amounts of juice over each fillet. Then drizzle each fillet with ½ tsp (2 mL) olive oil.
3. In a small bowl, combine sea salt, rosemary and dill. Sprinkle equally over fillets. Top each fillet with 2 lemon slices, 2 to 3 peppercorns, if using, and ¼ tsp (1 mL) butter.
4. Wrap foil tightly around each fillet by folding in two sides, then bringing top and bottom ends together in the center. Roll ends together, gently pressing out any air. Seal tightly.
5. Place sealed packets directly on oven rack. Bake in preheated oven for 15 minutes for 1-inch (2.5 cm) thick fillets; cooking time will vary depending on the thickness of the fish. Check the thinnest piece first: you want the fish to be just opaque and flaky. If necessary, reseal packet and return to oven for up to 7 minutes longer. Do not overcook!

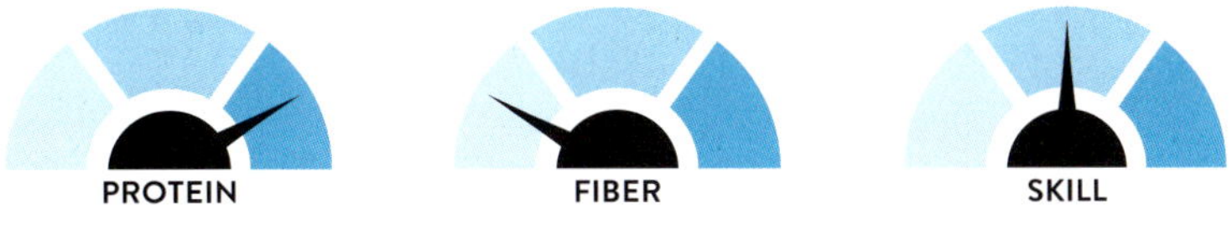


**NUTRIENTS PER SERVING**

| | | | | | |
|---|---|---|---|---|---|
| Calories | 310 kcal | Sodium | 470 mg | Vitamin D | 20 mcg |
| Fat | 19 g | Carbohydrate | 2 g | Calcium | 50 mg |
| Saturated fat | 6 g | Fiber | 1 g | Iron | 1 mg |
| Cholesterol | 80 mg | Protein | 30 g | Potassium | 628 mg |

# Smoky Salmon Bowl

- HIGH CALORIE
- MEDITERRANEAN DIET

**MAKES 6 SERVINGS**

**SERVING SIZE: 1 BOWL**

Salmon is full of omega-3 fatty acids, which are essential for brain health and cell protection. They also provide vitamin D, which is important for bone strength. This recipe also includes avocado, which provides healthy unsaturated fats. All of these nutrients combined make for a balanced, high-calorie dinner that is relatively easy to prepare.

### TIP

Check avocado ripeness by removing the stem cap on the top. If the stem comes off easily, then it's ready for eating.

- Preheat oven to 425°F (220°C)

| | | |
|---|---|---|
| 2 tbsp | store-bought taco seasoning mix | 30 mL |
| 2 tbsp | canola oil | 30 mL |
| 6 | salmon fillets (about 4 oz/125 g each) | 6 |
| 3 cups | hot cooked white or brown rice | 750 mL |
| 2 | avocados, peeled and sliced | 2 |
| 1 | can (19 oz/540 mL) black beans, drained and rinsed | 1 |
| 1½ cups | corn kernels | 375 mL |
| 1 cup | shredded red cabbage | 250 mL |
| 1 | lime, cut into wedges | 1 |
| | Chopped fresh cilantro or green onions | |
| | Salsa or sour cream | |

1. In a small bowl, stir together taco seasoning and oil.
2. Line a baking sheet with parchment paper and place salmon on top. Spread seasoning mixture all over salmon fillets. Roast in preheated oven for 10 minutes, or until fish flakes when tested.
3. Divide rice, avocados, beans, corn, cabbage and lime among six bowls, then top with salmon, cilantro and salsa.

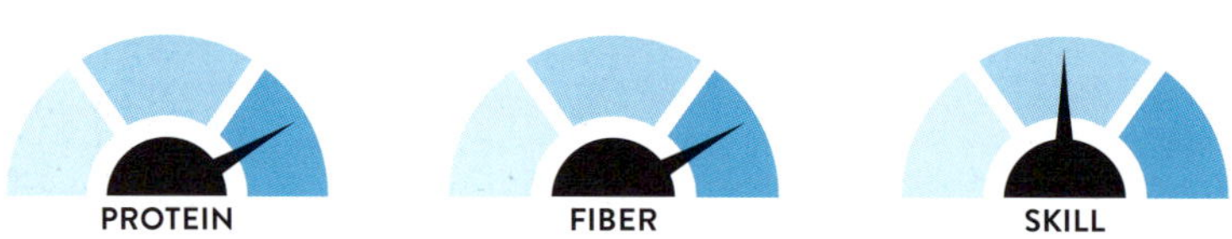


**NUTRIENTS PER SERVING**

| | | | | | |
|---|---|---|---|---|---|
| Calories | 544 kcal | Sodium | 1,193 mg | Vitamin D | 15 mcg |
| Fat | 24 g | Carbohydrate | 45 g | Calcium | 71 mg |
| Saturated fat | 3 g | Fiber | 10 g | Iron | 3 mg |
| Cholesterol | 64 mg | Protein | 3 g | Potassium | 946 mg |

# Almond Crusted Snapper

- HIGH CALORIE
- KETOGENIC DIET
- LOW CARBOHYDRATE
- MEDITERRANEAN DIET
- MIND DIET

**MAKES 4 SERVINGS**

**SERVING SIZE:**
**6 OZ (175 G)**

Snapper is a lean fish that is high in protein and B vitamins, which are essential for cellular energy production. Serve on a bed of rice and add a side salad for a balanced dinner.

### TIP

Substitute the snapper for any flaky white fish like grouper, pollack or tilapia.

- Preheat oven to 375°F (190°F)
- Food processor
- Baking sheet, coated with nonstick cooking spray

| | | |
|---|---|---|
| 1 cup | raw unsalted almonds, roughly chopped | 250 mL |
| 1/2 cup | fresh parsley, roughly chopped | 125 mL |
| 1/4 cup | extra-virgin olive oil | 60 mL |
| 4 | cloves garlic, crushed | 4 |
| 2 tsp | Dijon mustard | 10 mL |
| | Salt and ground black pepper | |
| 1 1/2 lbs | red snapper, cut into 4 fillets | 750 g |

1. In a small skillet, heat the almonds over medium-low heat and cook for about 5 minutes until toasted. Transfer the almonds to a clean bowl and let cool for 5 minutes.
2. Add the cooled almonds to a food processor and pulse until it reaches a flour-like consistency. Add the parsley, olive oil, garlic, mustard, 1/8 tsp (0.5 mL) salt and 1/8 tsp (0.5 mL) pepper and pulse until a paste forms.
3. Place the snapper fillets skin-side down onto the prepared baking sheet. Sprinkle 1/8 tsp (0.5 mL) salt and 1/8 tsp (0.5 mL) pepper over the snapper. Divide the almond paste equally among the fillets and, using clean hands, gently press to spread over the tops.
4. Bake until the snapper easily flakes with a fork, about 12 minutes. Serve warm.

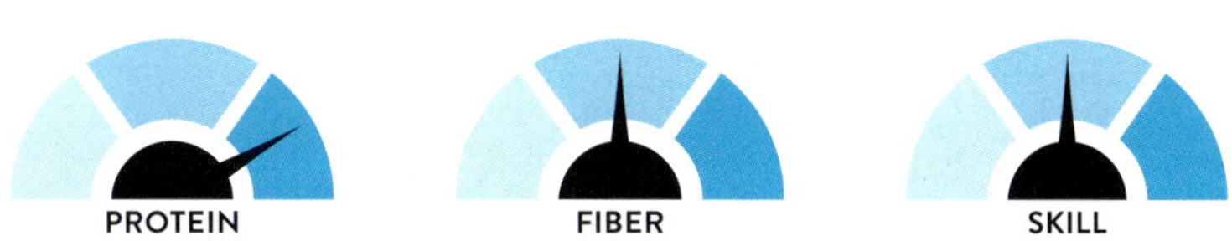


**NUTRIENTS PER SERVING**

| | | | | | |
|---|---|---|---|---|---|
| Calories | 614 kcal | Sodium | 348 mg | Vitamin D | 0 mcg |
| Fat | 45 g | Carbohydrate | 11 g | Calcium | 145 mg |
| Saturated fat | 6 g | Fiber | 6 g | Iron | 3 mg |
| Cholesterol | 74 mg | Protein | 45 g | Potassium | 441 mg |

# Stuffed Trout with Lemon Parsley Butter

- HIGH CALORIE
- KETOGENIC DIET
- LOW CARBOHYDRATE

**MAKES 4 SERVINGS**

Substitute olive oil instead of butter for a Mediterranean-forward option. Pair with a whole grain, such as brown rice, and a variety of vegetables for a balanced meal.

### TIP

If your trout fillets are large, you will need only 2; cut them in half to put them together.

| | | |
|---|---|---|
| 4 | trout fillets, skinless | 4 |
| 1 tsp | Montreal steak spice | 5 mL |
| 1 cup | store-bought artichoke and asiago dip | 250 mL |
| 1 | small shallot, finely diced | 1 |
| 1 | small red bell pepper, diced | 1 |
| 1/4 cup | butter, melted | 60 mL |
| 1/2 tsp | grated lemon zest | 2 mL |
| 2 tbsp | chopped fresh parsley | 30 mL |

1. Preheat oven to 425°F (220°C). Line a baking sheet with parchment paper.
2. Sprinkle trout fillets with steak spice all over and place 2 on prepared baking sheet. Divide and spread artichoke and asiago dip on the 2 fillets. Sprinkle with shallot and red pepper. Place remaining 2 trout fillets on top and press together gently.
3. Whisk together butter, lemon zest and parsley. Spoon overtop of trout fillets and bake for about 15 minutes or until trout flakes when tested with a fork.
4. Cut each stuffed trout in half to serve.

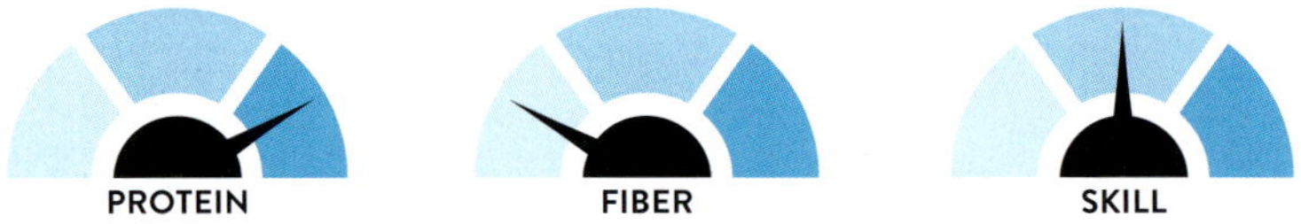


**NUTRIENTS PER SERVING**

| | | | | | |
|---|---|---|---|---|---|
| Calories | 550 kcal | Sodium | 780 mg | Vitamin D | 0 mcg |
| Fat | 40 g | Carbohydrate | 4 g | Calcium | 119 mg |
| Saturated fat | 15 g | Fiber | 0 g | Iron | 1 mg |
| Cholesterol | 250 mg | Protein | 43 g | Potassium | 949 mg |

# Skillet Gnocchi and Shrimp

- LOW CARBOHYDRATE
- MEDITERRANEAN DIET

**MAKES 4 SERVINGS**

One-skillet meals like this one save time when it comes to cleaning up after cooking. This also prevents having to move hot pots and pans around as much if oven safety is a concern.

| | | |
|---|---|---|
| **2 tbsp** | **extra-virgin olive oil** | **30 mL** |
| **1** | **package (12.5 oz/350 g) potato gnocchi** | **1** |
| **1** | **bag (12 oz/340 g) large black tiger shrimp, thawed, peeled and deveined** | **1** |
| **1** | **small zucchini, sliced into half moons** | **1** |
| **1⁄4 tsp** | **salt** | **1 mL** |
| **1⁄4 tsp** | **ground black pepper** | **1 mL** |
| **1⁄3 cup** | **sun-dried tomato pesto** | **75 mL** |

1. In a large nonstick skillet, heat oil over medium-high heat. Add gnocchi and sauté for about 5 minutes or until golden. Transfer with a slotted spoon to a bowl.
2. Return skillet to medium-high heat and sauté shrimp, zucchini, salt and pepper for about 5 minutes or until shrimp are pink and zucchini is golden. Reduce heat to medium and stir in gnocchi and pesto. Cook, stirring frequently, for about 2 minutes or until gnocchi are heated through.

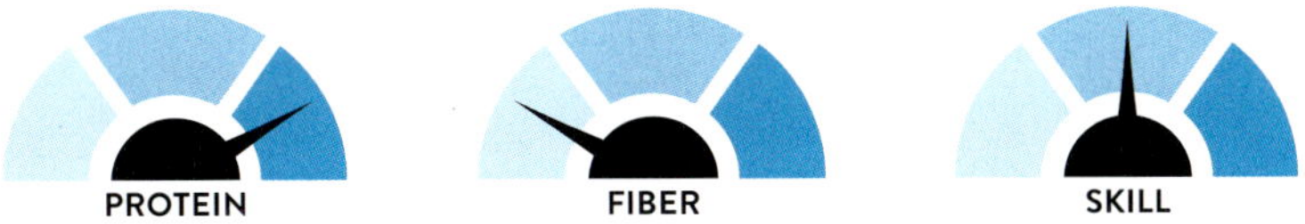


**NUTRIENTS PER SERVING**

| | | | | | |
|---|---|---|---|---|---|
| Calories | 330 kcal | Sodium | 760 mg | Vitamin D | 0 mcg |
| Fat | 16 g | Carbohydrate | 20 g | Calcium | 103 mg |
| Saturated fat | 5 g | Fiber | 2 g | Iron | 2 mg |
| Cholesterol | 145 mg | Protein | 21 g | Potassium | 283 mg |

# Cajun Shrimp and Rice Casserole

**MAKES 8 SERVINGS**

This recipe is a great use of whole grains (wild rice and brown rice)! Choose a gluten-free condensed soup for a gluten-free version.

### TIPS

The wild rice adds flavor and texture to this recipe, but it can also be made with white rice alone.

If your skillet isn't big enough to hold all of the ingredients, transfer the shrimp mixture to a large bowl once the cheese is melted.

- Preheat oven to 350°F (180°C)
- 13- by 9-inch (33 by 23 cm) glass baking dish, greased

| | | |
|---|---|---|
| 2 tsp | olive oil | 10 mL |
| 1 cup | chopped onion | 250 mL |
| 1 cup | chopped green bell pepper | 250 mL |
| 2 lbs | cooked medium shrimp | 1 kg |
| 4 oz | light pasteurized prepared cheese product, such as Velveeta, cubed | 125 g |
| 6 oz | light garlic-and-herb-flavored spreadable cheese, such as Boursin | 175 g |
| 1 | can (10 oz/284 mL) reduced-sodium, fat-free condensed cream of mushroom soup | 1 |
| 3 cups | cooked wild rice | 750 mL |
| 2 cups | cooked long-grain brown rice | 500 mL |
| 1 cup | chopped green onions | 250 mL |
| ½ tsp | salt | 2 mL |
| ¼ tsp | ground black pepper | 1 mL |

1. In a large nonstick skillet, heat oil over medium heat. Sauté onion and green pepper for 5 to 7 minutes or until softened. Add shrimp, pasteurized cheese, spreadable cheese and soup and cook, stirring occasionally, until cheese is melted. Stir in wild rice, brown rice, green onions, salt and pepper. Spoon into prepared baking dish.
2. Bake in preheated oven for 30 to 35 minutes or until bubbling.

PROTEIN

FIBER

SKILL

**NUTRIENTS PER SERVING**

| | | | | | |
|---|---|---|---|---|---|
| Calories | 440 kcal | Sodium | 1,130 mg | Vitamin D | 0 mcg |
| Fat | 20 g | Carbohydrate | 36 g | Calcium | 169 mg |
| Saturated fat | 9 g | Fiber | 3 g | Iron | 2 mg |
| Cholesterol | 205 mg | Protein | 27 g | Potassium | 471 mg |

# BBQ Tarragon Mustard Turkey

▶ LOW CARBOHYDRATE

**MAKES 6 SERVINGS**

Using a unique blend of flavors, this recipe offers a high-protein main to support muscle health. Pair with a side of vegetables and a whole grain for a balanced meal. Serve with rice pilaf, mixed baby summer squash and a spinach salad.

### TIP

Do not overcook the turkey or it may become dry. Check the temperature after 35 minutes, as barbecue temperatures can vary.

- Preheat greased barbecue grill to medium

| | | |
|---|---|---|
| 2 | cloves garlic, finely minced | 2 |
| 2 tsp | dried tarragon | 10 mL |
| ½ tsp | salt (optional) | 2 mL |
| ½ tsp | ground black pepper | 2 mL |
| 2 tbsp | Dijon mustard | 30 mL |
| 2 tbsp | chicken broth | 30 mL |
| 1 tbsp | canola oil, divided | 15 mL |
| 1 | bone-in skin-on turkey breast (about 2 lbs/1 kg) (see Tip, at left) | 1 |

1. In a small bowl, combine garlic, tarragon, salt (if using), pepper, mustard, broth and 2 tsp (10 mL) of the oil.
2. Gently loosen and raise the skin of the turkey breast, but do not remove it. Spread the garlic mixture evenly on the meat under the skin and replace the skin. Spread the remaining oil over the skin.
3. Place turkey, skin side down, on preheated grill. Close lid and grill for 10 minutes. Turn breast over so skin side is up, close lid and grill for 40 to 45 minutes or until no longer pink inside and a meat thermometer inserted in the thickest part registers 170°F (77°C). Transfer to a cutting board, tent with foil and let rest for 10 minutes before slicing.

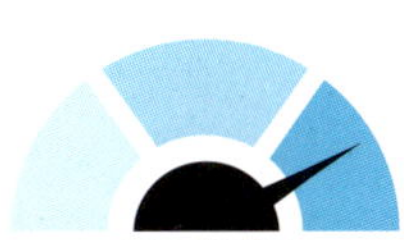
PROTEIN

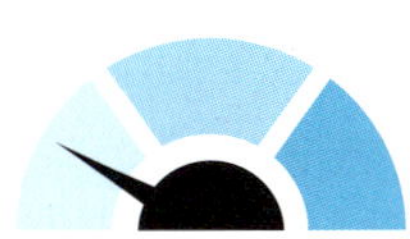
FIBER

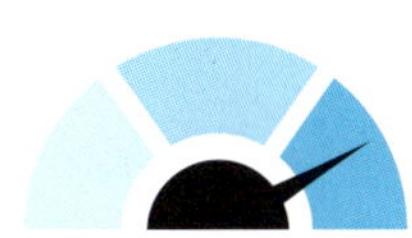
SKILL

**NUTRIENTS PER SERVING**

| | | | | | |
|---|---|---|---|---|---|
| Calories | 200 kcal | Sodium | 450 mg | Vitamin D | 0 mcg |
| Fat | 5 g | Carbohydrate | 1 g | Calcium | 25 mg |
| Saturated fat | 1 g | Fiber | 0 g | Iron | 1 mg |
| Cholesterol | 85 mg | Protein | 36 g | Potassium | 389 mg |

# Sweet Potato Chicken Chili

- HIGH CALORIE
- MEDITERRANEAN DIET

**MAKES 4 SERVINGS**

**SERVING SIZE: ABOUT 2 CUPS (500 ML)**

This hearty meal combines sweet potatoes and black beans for a high-fiber twist on a classic comfort food.

| | | |
|---|---|---|
| 2 tbsp | extra-virgin olive oil or canola oil | 30 mL |
| 1 | small yellow onion, diced | 1 |
| 1½ lbs | sweet potatoes, peeled and cut into ½-inch (1 cm) cubes (4 cups/1 L) (see Tip, opposite) | 750 g |
| 1 tbsp | chili powder | 15 mL |
| 2 tsp | ground cumin | 10 mL |
| 1 tsp | smoked paprika | 5 mL |
| ½ tsp | salt | 2 mL |
| ¼ tsp | ground black pepper | 1 mL |
| ⅛ tsp | ground cinnamon | 0.5 mL |
| 1 | can (28 oz/796 mL) crushed tomatoes, with juice | 1 |
| 1 cup | reduced-sodium chicken broth | 250 mL |
| 15 oz | frozen corn kernels, thawed | 425 g |
| 1 | can (14- to 19-oz/398 to 540 mL) reduced-sodium black beans, drained and rinsed | 1 |
| 2 cups | coarsely chopped rotisserie chicken | 500 mL |

1. Heat the oil in a large saucepan over medium heat. When the oil is shimmering, add the onion and sauté until soft and translucent, 3 minutes.

PROTEIN

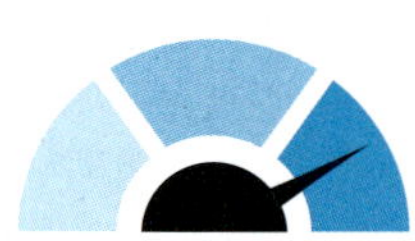
FIBER

SKILL

**NUTRIENTS PER SERVING**

| | | | | | |
|---|---|---|---|---|---|
| Calories | 643 kcal | Sodium | 1,283 mg | Vitamin D | 0 mcg |
| Fat | 17 g | Carbohydrate | 98 g | Calcium | 212 mg |
| Saturated fat | 3 g | Fiber | 22 g | Iron | 9 mg |
| Cholesterol | 76 mg | Protein | 35 g | Potassium | 2,107 mg |

**TIP**

When selecting sweet potatoes, choose those that are firm, with intact skin and without blemishes or large dents. Store in a cool, dry place for up to 1 month.

2. Add the sweet potatoes, chili powder, cumin, paprika, salt, pepper and cinnamon and toss to combine. Cook, stirring occasionally, until the mixture is fragrant, 1 to 2 minutes. Stir in the crushed tomatoes with juice, chicken broth, corn and beans. Increase the heat to high and bring the mixture to a boil. Decrease the heat to medium-low, cover and simmer, stirring occasionally, until the potatoes are tender and the mixture has thickened, about 25 minutes.

3. Add the chicken, increase the heat to high and bring to a boil. Decrease the heat to medium and cook, uncovered, stirring occasionally, until the chicken is heated through, about 3 minutes.

# Chicken Stir-Fry with Red Peppers, Broccoli and Walnuts

- HIGH CALORIE
- MEDITERRANEAN DIET

**MAKES 4 SERVINGS**

**SERVING SIZE: ABOUT 2 CUPS (500 ML) STIR-FRY PLUS ½ CUP (125 ML) RICE**

A complete meal — no need for additional sides! Quality features include the use of whole grains, nuts, vegetables and olive oil — all key components of the Mediterranean diet.

| | | |
|---|---|---|
| 1 cup | long-grain brown rice | 250 mL |
| 2¼ cups | low-sodium chicken broth, divided | 560 mL |
| 2 tbsp | reduced-sodium soy sauce | 30 mL |
| 1 tbsp | unseasoned rice vinegar | 15 mL |
| 2 tsp | cornstarch | 10 mL |
| 1 tsp | liquid honey | 5 mL |
| 1 tsp | freshly squeezed lime juice | 5 mL |
| ¼ tsp | ground ginger | 1 mL |
| 1 lb | boneless skinless chicken breasts, cut into 1-inch (2.5 cm) cubes | 500 g |
| ¼ tsp | salt | 1 mL |
| ⅛ tsp | ground black pepper | 0.5 mL |
| 3 tbsp | olive oil, divided | 45 mL |
| 2 | red bell peppers, cut into ½-inch (1 cm) strips | 2 |
| 4 cups | broccoli florets | 1 L |
| ¼ cup | coarsely chopped raw walnuts | 60 mL |

1. In a medium saucepan, bring the rice and 2 cups (500 mL) of the broth to a boil over high heat. Reduce the heat to low and simmer, covered, until the broth is absorbed, 35 to 40 minutes. Fluff the rice with a fork.
2. In a small bowl, whisk together the remaining ¼ cup (60 mL) broth, soy sauce, rice vinegar, cornstarch, honey, lime juice and ground ginger.

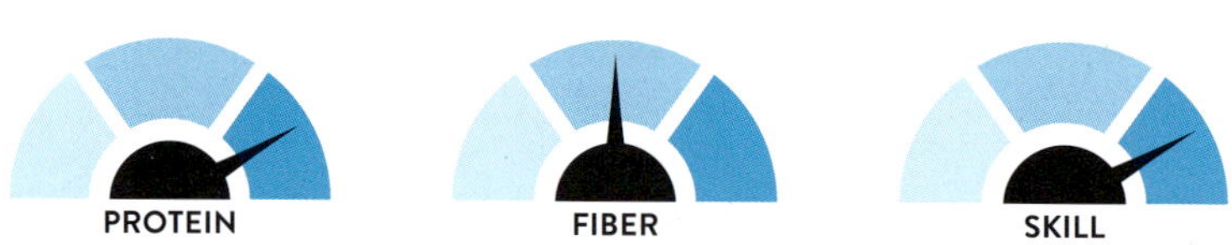


**NUTRIENTS PER SERVING**

| | | | | | |
|---|---|---|---|---|---|
| Calories | 523 kcal | Sodium | 574 mg | Vitamin D | 1 mcg |
| Fat | 20 g | Carbohydrate | 49 g | Calcium | 71 mg |
| Saturated fat | 3 g | Fiber | 5 g | Iron | 1 mg |
| Cholesterol | 86 mg | Protein | 35 g | Potassium | 1,034 mg |

**TIP**

The chicken in this recipe provides a quality source of lean protein. Protein is important for muscle maintenance, especially for those losing weight. When cooking with chicken, be sure to remove the skin to reduce your intake of saturated fats.

3. Sprinkle both sides of the chicken with the salt and black pepper. In a large skillet or wok, heat 2 tbsp (30 mL) of the oil over medium heat. When the oil is shimmering, add the chicken and cook on all sides until an instant-read thermometer registers 165°F (74°C), about 8 minutes. Transfer the chicken to a clean plate.

4. Heat the remaining 1 tbsp (15 mL) oil in the same skillet or wok. When the oil is shimmering, add the red peppers and broccoli and cook until slightly softened, about 5 minutes. Add the broth mixture, increase the heat to high and bring to a boil, then reduce the heat to medium and cook until the sauce is slightly thickened, 1 minute. Add the chicken back into the skillet or wok and toss to evenly coat with the sauce. Sprinkle with the walnuts.

5. To serve, divide the rice among four plates and top with the chicken stir-fry. Serve warm.

# Coconut Chicken with Quinoa

**MAKES 4 SERVINGS**

For less saturated fat, remove the chicken skin. Quinoa is a whole grain that provides all of the essential amino acids — meaning it has fiber, protein and lots of vitamins and minerals! This sustainable source of energy is a great addition to any meal to help promote stable energy levels throughout the day.

### TIP

If you prefer, you can substitute already-ground spices for the cumin seeds and allspice and skip the toasting step. I'd use 1 tsp (5 mL) ground cumin and ½ tsp (2 mL) ground allspice in this recipe.

| | | |
|---|---|---|
| 2 tsp | cumin seeds (see Tip, left) | 10 mL |
| 1 tsp | whole allspice (see Tip, left) | 5 mL |
| 1 tbsp | olive oil | 15 mL |
| 1½ lbs | skin-on bone-in chicken breasts, patted dry | 750 g |
| 1 | onion, finely chopped | 1 |
| 1 | red bell pepper, diced | 1 |
| 1 | green bell pepper, diced | 1 |
| 6 | cloves garlic, minced | 6 |
| ½ to 1 | chile pepper, seeded and minced, optional | ½ to 1 |
| 1 tsp | curry powder | 5 mL |
| ½ tsp | salt | 2 mL |
| ½ tsp | ground black pepper | 2 mL |
| ¾ cup | quinoa, rinsed and drained | 175 mL |
| 1½ cups | reduced-sodium chicken stock | 375 mL |
| ½ cup | coconut milk | 125 mL |

1. In a dry large skillet with lid over medium heat, combine cumin seeds and allspice. Toast, stirring constantly, until fragrant, about 4 minutes. Immediately transfer to a mortar or a spice grinder and grind. Set aside.

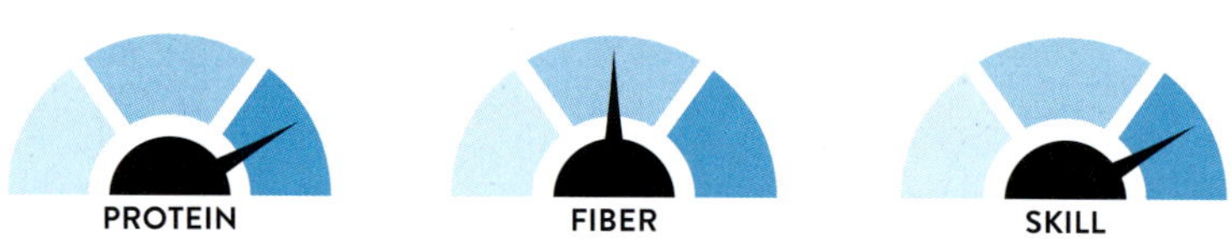


**NUTRIENTS PER SERVING**

| | | | | | |
|---|---|---|---|---|---|
| Calories | 342 kcal | Sodium | 558 mg | Vitamin D | 0 mg |
| Fat | 9 g | Carbohydrate | 32 g | Calcium | 118 mg |
| Saturated fat | 2 g | Fiber | 5 g | Iron | 3 mg |
| Cholesterol | 86 mg | Protein | 32 g | Potassium | 886 mg |

**NUTRIENT TIP**

The crispy chicken skin adds texture and flavor to this dish, but it also adds fat. If you want to reduce the quantity of fat, remove the skin. Most of the saturated fat comes from the chicken skin and the coconut milk.

2. In same skillet, heat oil over medium heat for 30 seconds. Add chicken, in batches, skin side down, and brown well, about 4 minutes. Turn over, cover and cook for 10 minutes. Remove from pan and keep warm. Drain all but 1 tbsp (15 mL) fat from pan.

3. Add onion, red pepper, green pepper, garlic and chile pepper, if using, and cook, stirring, until vegetables are softened, about 5 minutes. Add curry powder, salt, black pepper, reserved ground spices and quinoa and cook, stirring, until quinoa is well integrated into mixture, about 1 minute. Add stock and coconut milk and bring to a boil. Lay chicken, skin side up, over mixture. Reduce heat to low. Cover and cook until chicken is no longer pink inside, about 30 minutes.

# Herbed Turkey Chickpea Meatballs with Yogurt Sauce

- ◗ DYSPHAGIA-FRIENDLY
- ◗ MEDITERRANEAN DIET

**MAKES 6 SERVINGS**

**SERVING SIZE: 5 MEATBALLS PLUS ¼ CUP (60 ML) SAUCE**

This unique take on meatballs combines a lean animal protein with a fiber-rich plant-based protein, providing a variety of vitamins and minerals essential for overall health. Add a side of raw cucumber or carrots for even more nutrients!

- Preheat the oven to 375°F (190°C).
- Food processor or blender
- 2 baking sheets, coated with nonstick cooking spray

### *Sauce*

| | | |
|---|---|---|
| 1½ cups | plain nonfat Greek yogurt | 375 mL |
| | Zest and juice of 1 lemon | |
| ¼ cup | chopped fresh parsley | 60 mL |
| 2 | cloves garlic, minced | 2 |
| ¼ tsp | salt | 1 mL |
| ⅛ tsp | ground black pepper | 0.5 mL |

### *Meatballs*

| | | |
|---|---|---|
| 1 | can (14- to 19-oz/398 to 540 mL) low-sodium chickpeas, drained and rinsed | 1 |
| 1 | yellow onion, halved and thinly sliced | 1 |
| | Juice of 1 lemon | |
| ¼ cup | fresh parsley | 60 mL |
| 1 | large egg | 1 |
| 2 | cloves garlic, crushed | 2 |
| ½ tsp | smoked paprika | 2 mL |
| ½ tsp | salt | 2 mL |
| ⅛ tsp | ground black pepper | 0.5 mL |
| 1 lb | lean ground turkey | 500 g |
| ½ cup | dry unseasoned bread crumbs | 125 mL |
| ¼ cup | extra-virgin olive oil, divided | 60 mL |

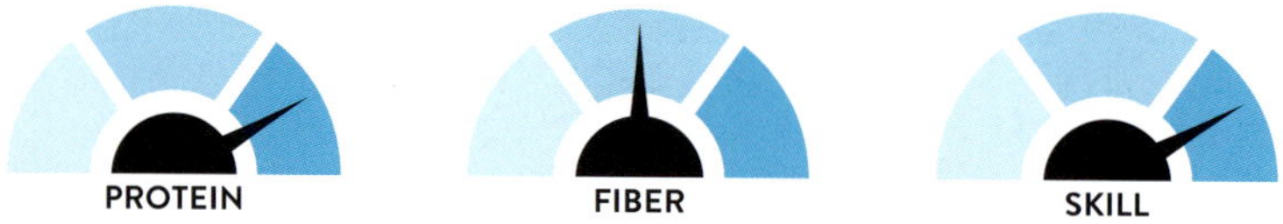


**NUTRIENTS PER SERVING**

| | | | | | |
|---|---|---|---|---|---|
| Calories | 370 kcal | Sodium | 510 mg | Vitamin D | 24 mcg |
| Fat | 12 g | Carbohydrate | 34 g | Calcium | 118 mg |
| Saturated fat | 2 g | Fiber | 5 g | Iron | 3 mg |
| Cholesterol | 70 mg | Protein | 31 g | Potassium | 517 mg |

**TIP**

Replace the parsley with the same amount of cilantro or dill, or use a different fresh herb of your choice.

1. **Make the sauce:** In a medium bowl, whisk together the yogurt, lemon zest and juice, parsley, garlic, salt and pepper until combined. Cover and place in the refrigerator to let the flavors combine for at least 20 minutes and up to 5 days.

2. **Make the meatballs:** In the bowl of the food processor or blender, add the chickpeas, onion, lemon juice, parsley, egg, garlic, smoked paprika, salt and pepper. Process or blend on High until well combined, about 1 minute.

3. Transfer the chickpea mixture to a large mixing bowl. Add the turkey and bread crumbs and stir to combine.

4. Using clean hands, scoop 1 heaping tbsp (15 mL) of the turkey-chickpea mixture and roll into a ball. Place on a clean plate and repeat, keeping meatballs about ½ inch (1 cm) apart. You should have a total of 30 meatballs. Cover and refrigerate for at least 30 minutes.

5. Preheat the oven to 375°F (190°C).

6. In a large skillet, heat 2 tbsp (30 mL) of the oil over medium heat. When the oil is shimmering, add half of the meatballs and cook, browning all sides, about 6 minutes. Transfer to one of the prepared baking sheets, leaving 1 inch (2.5 cm) between meatballs. Repeat with the remaining oil, meatballs and prepared baking sheet.

7. Bake until the meatballs are golden brown and fully cooked through, 15 to 18 minutes. Remove the baking sheets from the oven and let the meatballs cool for 10 minutes. Repeat with the remaining oil, meatballs and prepared baking sheet.

8. To serve, divide the meatballs among six plates and serve with ¼ cup (60 mL) of the yogurt sauce on the side.

# Sheet-Pan Chicken Shawarma

**MEDITERRANEAN DIET**

**MAKES 6 SERVINGS**

**SERVING SIZE: 1 PITA SANDWICH**

The perfect sheet-pan meal to save time and energy. This recipe uses lean protein and lots of spices. Choose low-fat yogurt and olive oil to adhere more closely to a Mediterranean diet. Add even more vegetables for an extra boost of fiber, vitamins and minerals!

- Preheat oven to 425°F (220°C)
- Large rimmed baking sheet

| | | |
|---|---|---|
| ½ cup | plain yogurt | 125 mL |
| 5 | cloves garlic, minced | 5 |
| 1 tbsp | smoked paprika | 15 mL |
| 1½ tsp | salt | 7 mL |
| 1 tsp | ground coriander | 5 mL |
| 1 tsp | ground cumin | 5 mL |
| 1 tsp | ground turmeric | 5 mL |
| 1 tsp | ground cinnamon | 5 mL |
| 1 tsp | ground cardamom | 5 mL |
| 1½ lbs | boneless skinless chicken thighs, sliced into 1-inch (2.5 cm) strips | 750 g |
| 2 tbsp | canola oil, divided | 30 mL |
| 1 | red bell pepper, sliced | 1 |
| 1 | yellow bell pepper, sliced | 1 |
| 1 | onion, thinly sliced | 1 |
| | Hummus | |
| 6 | pita bread | 6 |

1. Place one oven rack in the middle position and another about 5 inches (12.5 cm) below the broiler.

2. In a large bowl, combine yogurt, garlic, paprika, salt, coriander, cumin, turmeric, cinnamon and cardamom. Add chicken and stir until evenly coated. Marinate 15 minutes.

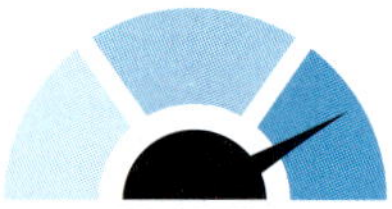
PROTEIN

FIBER

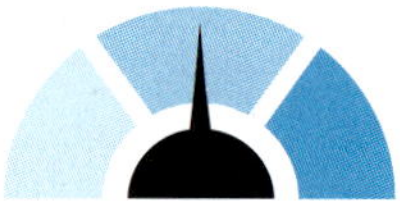
SKILL

**NUTRIENTS PER SERVING**

| | | | | | |
|---|---|---|---|---|---|
| Calories | 400 kcal | Sodium | 1,260 mg | Vitamin D | 0 mcg |
| Fat | 16 g | Carbohydrate | 43 g | Calcium | 173 mg |
| Saturated fat | 3 g | Fiber | 2 g | Iron | 4 mg |
| Cholesterol | 95 mg | Protein | 30 g | Potassium | 287 mg |

### TIPS

Line the baking sheet with foil for easier cleanup.

Try other flatbread options, such as balady, naan, tortilla or lavash.

3. Drizzle rimmed baking sheet with 1 tbsp (15 mL) of the oil, then arrange chicken, red pepper, yellow pepper and onion in an even layer, then drizzle with remaining oil. Bake on the middle rack, stirring ingredients halfway through cooking time, for 12 minutes or until chicken is cooked through. Turn on broiler, move baking sheet to top rack and broil 3 minutes or until meat and vegetables are slightly charred.

4. Spread a generous portion of hummus on each pita bread, then add chicken and roasted vegetables along with plenty of suggested toppings. Fold up and eat with your hands.

# Sunday Pot Roast with Cumin-Spiked Barley

- DYSPHAGIA-FRIENDLY
- LOW CARBOHYDRATE
- MEDITERRANEAN DIET

**MAKES 8 SERVINGS**

The use of extra virgin olive oil, whole grains, herbs and spices makes this a fun Mediterranean twist on a household classic. It's a prime example of how a small amount of red meat can be incorporated into a Mediterranean diet. Slow cooker recipes come in handy when you don't have much time or energy to cook. Slow cooking also makes food softer and easier to chew for those with chewing and swallowing difficulty.

- Works best in a large (minimum 5-quart) slow cooker

| | | |
|---|---|---|
| 1/4 cup | all-purpose flour | 60 mL |
| 1 tsp | dried thyme | 5 mL |
| | Salt | |
| | Ground black pepper | |
| 3 lbs | boneless beef pot roast | 1.5 kg |
| 1 tbsp | olive oil (approx.) | 15 mL |
| 2 | onions, finely chopped | 2 |
| 3 | carrots, peeled and diced | 3 |
| 4 | stalks celery, diced | 4 |
| 4 | cloves garlic, minced | 4 |
| 1 | bay leaf | 1 |
| 2 tbsp | ground cumin | 30 mL |
| 1 cup | barley (see Tips, opposite), rinsed and drained | 250 mL |
| 2 cups | water | 500 mL |
| 2 cups | beef stock | 500 mL |
| 1 cup | dry red wine | 250 mL |
| 1/2 cup | chopped fresh parsley | 125 mL |

1. On a plate, combine flour, 1/2 tsp (2 mL) thyme, 1/2 tsp (2 mL) salt and pepper. Dredge roast, covering all sides, and set any remaining flour mixture aside.
2. In a large skillet, heat 1 tbsp (15 mL) oil over medium heat for 30 seconds. Add roast and brown on all sides, about 8 minutes. Transfer to slow cooker stoneware.

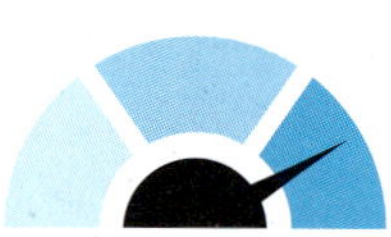
PROTEIN

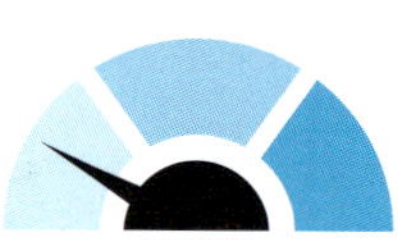
FIBER

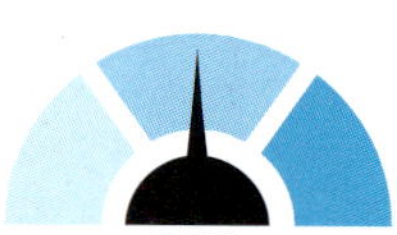
SKILL

**NUTRIENTS PER SERVING**

| | | | | | |
|---|---|---|---|---|---|
| Calories | 385 kcal | Sodium | 1,030 mg | Vitamin D | 0 mcg |
| Fat | 10 g | Carbohydrate | 18 g | Calcium | 653 mg |
| Saturated fat | 3 g | Fiber | 3 g | Iron | 8 mg |
| Cholesterol | 131 mg | Protein | 52 g | Potassium | 653 mg |

## TIPS

For the best flavor, toast and grind whole cumin seeds rather than buying ground cumin. Simply stir seeds in a dry skillet over medium heat until fragrant, about 3 minutes. Immediately transfer to a spice grinder or mortar and grind.

Use the variety of barley you prefer — pearled, pot or whole. Whole (also known as hulled) barley is the most nutritious form of the grain.

3. Add more oil to pan, if necessary. Add onions, carrots and celery; cook, stirring, until softened, about 7 minutes. Add garlic, bay leaf and cumin; cook, stirring, for 1 minute. Add reserved flour mixture and cook, stirring, for 1 minute. Add barley and toss to coat. Add water, stock and wine; bring to a boil. Pour over roast, making sure it thoroughly coats the meat.

4. Cover and cook on Low for 10 hours or on High for 5 hours, until meat is very tender. Discard bay leaf. Taste and add salt and pepper, if necessary.

5. Transfer meat to a deep platter or serving dish and slice thinly. Cover with sauce and garnish with parsley.

# Pork Chop and Veggie Sheet-Pan Dinner

**MAKES 4 SERVINGS**

Sheet-pan dinners are an easy way to make meals without the added clean up. Simply combine everything on a sheet pan and pop it in the oven for a quick and effortless dinner.

### TIPS

Look for pork chops about ¾ inch (2 cm) thick for a great juicy chop.

Substitute a red bell pepper for the onion for a change in flavor.

- Preheat oven to 425°F (220° C)
- Rimmed baking sheet, lined with parchment paper

| | | |
|---|---|---|
| 1 lb | mini potatoes, halved | 500 g |
| 1 | bag (12 oz/375 g) baby carrots | 1 |
| 1 | small red onion, cut into wedges | 1 |
| 3 | garlic cloves, minced | 3 |
| 2 tbsp | canola oil | 30 mL |
| 2 tsp | chopped fresh rosemary | 10 mL |
| ½ tsp | each salt and black pepper, divided | 2 mL |
| 4 | pork loin boneless center-cut chops (about 1 lb/500 g total) | 4 |
| ¼ cup | barbecue sauce | 60 mL |
| 1 tbsp | chopped fresh parsley | 15 mL |

1. Spread potatoes, carrots, onion and garlic on prepared baking sheet. Drizzle with oil and sprinkle with rosemary and half each of the salt and pepper. Toss gently to coat. Roast for 10 minutes.
2. Meanwhile, toss pork chops with remaining salt and pepper. Add barbecue sauce and parsley; toss to coat well. Add pork chops to baking sheet and return to oven for 15 minutes or until pork is no longer pink inside and thermometer inserted in pork reaches 155°F (68°C).

PROTEIN

FIBER

SKILL

**NUTRIENTS PER SERVING**

| | | | | | |
|---|---|---|---|---|---|
| Calories | 370 kcal | Sodium | 860 mg | Vitamin D | 0 mcg |
| Fat | 16 g | Carbohydrate | 35 g | Calcium | 45 mg |
| Saturated fat | 4.5 g | Fiber | 6 g | Iron | 2 mg |
| Cholesterol | 60 mg | Protein | 24 g | Potassium | 1,267 mg |

# Lamb Shoulder Chops with Olives

- HIGH CALORIE
- KETOGENIC DIET
- LOW CARBOHYDRATE

**MAKES 4 SERVINGS**

**SERVING SIZE: 1 LAMB CHOP**

High in calories and protein, this dish is great for those trying to maintain or gain weight.

| | | |
|---|---|---|
| 4 | lamb shoulder chops (about 1½ lbs/750 g total) | 4 |
| ¼ tsp | salt | 1 mL |
| ¼ tsp | ground black pepper | 1 mL |
| 2 tbsp | canola oil | 30 mL |
| 2 | sprigs fresh rosemary | 2 |
| 2 | cloves garlic | 2 |
| ½ cup | dry white wine | 125 mL |
| ½ cup | pitted cracked green or small green olives | 125 mL |
| ½ | lemon | ½ |
| 2 tbsp | butter | 30 mL |
| 2 tbsp | chopped fresh parsley | 30 mL |

1. Sprinkle lamb chops with salt and pepper.
2. In a large nonstick skillet, heat oil, rosemary and garlic over medium-low heat. Cook, turning rosemary often, for about 5 minutes or until fragrant. Increase heat to medium-high heat, add lamb chops and brown both sides well. Transfer to a plate.
3. Reduce heat to medium and add wine; simmer for 1 minute. Add olives, squeeze lemon juice from lemon half into skillet, and add with butter. Return lamb chops to skillet and cook, turning occasionally, for about 8 minutes or until chops reach an internal temperature of 145°F (63°C) for medium-rare or until desired doneness. Garnish with the parsley and serve.

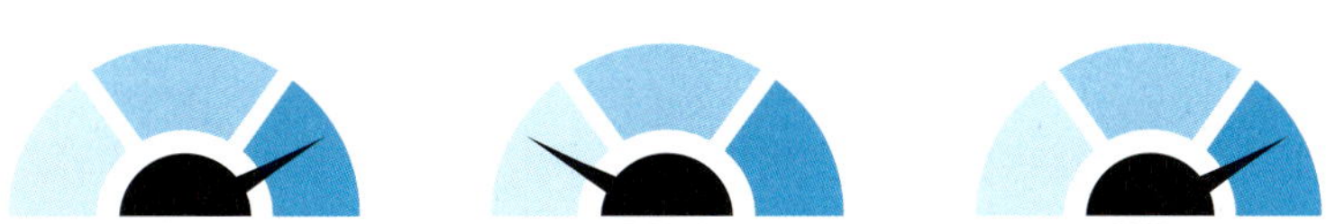


**NUTRIENTS PER SERVING**

| | | | | | |
|---|---|---|---|---|---|
| Calories | 590 kcal | Sodium | 770 mg | Vitamin D | 0 mcg |
| Fat | 35 g | Carbohydrate | 3 g | Calcium | 75 mg |
| Saturated fat | 12 g | Fiber | 1 g | Iron | 5 mg |
| Cholesterol | 205 mg | Protein | 59 g | Potassium | 555 mg |

## CHAPTER 14

# SNACKS AND SMOOTHIES

# Black Bean Salsa

▶ MEDITERRANEAN DIET

**MAKES 6 SERVINGS**

The combination of beans and vegetables in this recipe provides approximately half of the fiber you need in one day! This snack is sure to make you feel full and satisfied while supporting gut health.

## TIPS

Cover and refrigerate for up to 3 days. Stir well and season if necessary.

Cilantro lovers unite! If you love that fresh herb flavor, add double the amount of cilantro.

For a mango variation, peel, pit and dice 1 fresh ripe mango and stir into the black bean salsa. Adjust lime juice and salt to your taste.

| | | |
|---|---|---|
| 2 | cans (19 oz/540 mL each) black beans, drained and rinsed | 2 |
| ½ cup | diced tomato | 125 mL |
| ⅓ cup | chopped fresh cilantro | 75 mL |
| ¼ cup | diced red onion | 60 mL |
| 1 | jalapeño pepper, seeded and diced | 1 |
| 2 | cloves garlic, minced | 2 |
| ½ tsp | grated lime zest | 2 mL |
| 2 tbsp | freshly squeezed lime juice | 30 mL |
| 2 tbsp | canola oil | 30 mL |
| ½ tsp | salt | 2 mL |

1. In a large bowl, stir together beans, tomato, cilantro, onion, jalapeño, garlic, lime zest, lime juice, oil and salt. Let stand 10 minutes before serving.

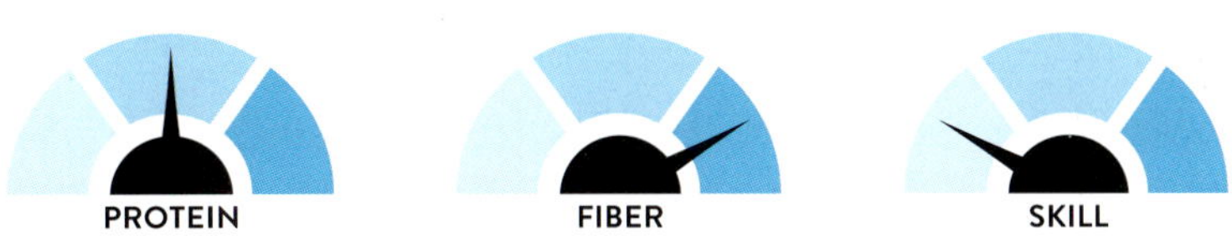


**NUTRIENTS PER SERVING**

| | | | | | |
|---|---|---|---|---|---|
| Calories | 271 kcal | Sodium | 534 mg | Vitamin D | 0 mcg |
| Fat | 6 g | Carbohydrate | 39 g | Calcium | 81 mg |
| Saturated fat | 0 g | Fiber | 16 g | Iron | 4 mg |
| Cholesterol | 0 mg | Protein | 13 g | Potassium | 739 mg |

# Holy Smokes Pita Chips

- MEDITERRANEAN DIET
- MIND DIET

**MAKES 48 WEDGES**

**SERVING SIZE: 4 WEDGES**

This is a great potato chip alternative that has less fat and more fiber. We recommend pairing with your favorite dip, such as hummus, guacamole or a Greek yogurt dip.

## TIPS

For ease in cutting, stack 2 to 3 pitas together before cutting them into wedges.

These chips will stay crisp in a sealable plastic bag or airtight container for up to 7 days.

- **Preheat oven to 375°F (190°C)**

| | | |
|---|---|---|
| 2 | cloves garlic, finely minced | 2 |
| 2 tsp | ground cumin | 10 mL |
| 1/2 tsp | chili powder | 2 mL |
| 1/2 tsp | paprika | 2 mL |
| 1/2 tsp | curry powder | 2 mL |
| 1/2 tsp | ground black pepper | 2 mL |
| 1/4 tsp | salt | 1 mL |
| 1 to 2 tbsp | canola oil | 15 to 30 mL |
| 2 to 3 | drops hot pepper sauce | 2 to 3 |
| 6 | 6-inch (15 cm) whole wheat pitas | 6 |

1. In a small bowl, combine garlic, cumin, chili powder, paprika, curry powder, black pepper, salt, oil and hot pepper sauce to taste.
2. Using a pastry brush, coat both sides of each pita with spice mixture and cut each into 8 wedges. Spread wedges in a single layer on two baking sheets.
3. Bake in preheated oven, turning once, for 8 to 10 minutes or until pitas are brown and crisp. Let cool completely on pans on a wire rack.

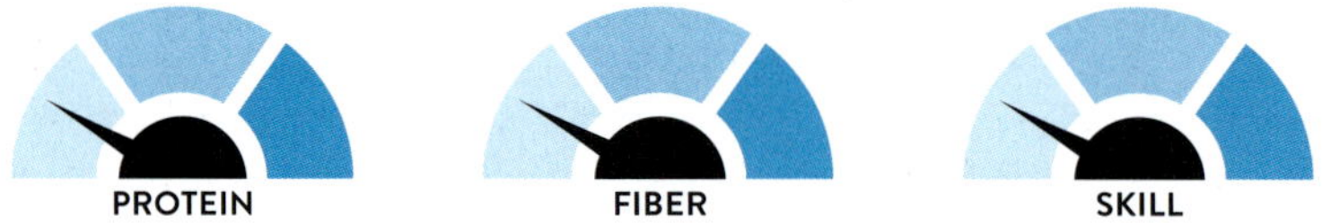


**NUTRIENTS PER SERVING**

| | | | | | |
|---|---|---|---|---|---|
| Calories | 108 kcal | Sodium | 221 mg | Vitamin D | 0 mcg |
| Fat | 3 g | Carbohydrate | 18 g | Calcium | 12 mg |
| Saturated fat | 0 g | Fiber | 2 g | Iron | 1 mg |
| Cholesterol | 0 mg | Protein | 3 g | Potassium | 72 mg |

# Edamame with Asian Vinaigrette

- KETOGENIC DIET
- LOW CARBOHYDRATE
- MEDITERRANEAN DIET

**MAKES ABOUT 3 CUPS (750 ML)**

**SERVING SIZE: ¾ CUP (175 ML)**

This is a higher-sodium snack — great for people looking to add salt to their diets to help with low blood pressure! To decrease the sodium in this recipe, opt for low-sodium soy sauce.

### TIP

Ginger is very easy to purée if kept whole in the freezer. Remove from the freezer as required and grate with skin on.

| | | |
|---|---|---|
| 12 cups | water | 3 L |
| 3 tbsp | salt | 45 mL |
| 3 cups | edamame in the pod, trimmed | 750 mL |
| ¼ cup | thinly sliced shallots | 60 mL |
| 1 tbsp | soy sauce | 15 mL |
| 2 tsp | rice vinegar | 10 mL |
| ½ tsp | chopped fresh cilantro leaves | 2 mL |
| ¼ tsp | puréed fresh gingerroot (see Tip, left) | 1 mL |
| ¼ tsp | toasted sesame oil | 1 mL |

1. In a saucepan, bring water and salt to a boil over high heat. Add edamame and boil until soybeans are tender-crisp and vibrant green, about 6 minutes.
2. Drain beans and transfer to a large bowl. Add shallots, soy sauce, vinegar, cilantro, ginger and sesame oil and toss to coat. Serve immediately or cover and refrigerate for up to 3 days.

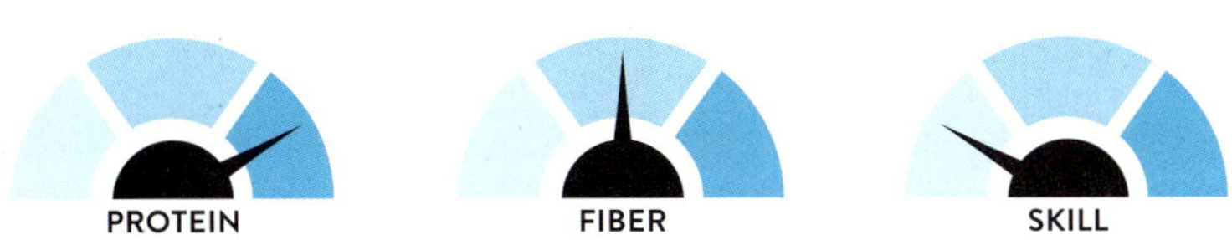


**NUTRIENTS PER SERVING**

| | | | | | |
|---|---|---|---|---|---|
| Calories | 144 kcal | Sodium | 812 mg | Vitamin D | 0 mcg |
| Fat | 6 g | Carbohydrate | 13 g | Calcium | 95 mg |
| Saturated fat | 0 g | Fiber | 6 g | Iron | 3 mg |
| Cholesterol | 0 mg | Protein | 14 g | Potassium | 667 mg |

# Hummus from Scratch

- DYSPHAGIA-FRIENDLY
- MEDITERRANEAN DIET
- MIND DIET

**MAKES ABOUT 3 CUPS (750 ML)**

**SERVING SIZE: 2 TBSP (30 ML)**

Full of flavor, this recipe is a great way to incorporate more plant-based protein. If you're in a crunch, buy low-sodium canned chickpeas and cook according to directions on the can. Serve with Holy Smokes Pita Chips (page 214) and fresh vegetables.

- Food processor

| | | |
|---|---|---|
| 1 cup | dried chickpeas (see Tips, opposite) | 250 mL |
| 1/3 cup | tahini | 75 mL |
| 1/3 cup | extra-virgin olive oil | 75 mL |
| 1/4 cup | freshly squeezed lemon juice (approx.) | 60 mL |
| 1/4 cup | flat-leaf (Italian) parsley leaves | 60 mL |
| 2 | cloves garlic (approx.) | 2 |
| 1 tsp | ground cumin | 5 mL |
| 1 tsp | salt (approx.) | 5 mL |
| 1/2 tsp | ground black pepper | 2 mL |
| 1/4 tsp | cayenne pepper (optional) | 1 mL |
| | Sweet paprika (optional) | |

1. In a large saucepan, combine chickpeas and 3 cups (750 mL) cold water. Set aside to soak for at least 6 hours or overnight. Drain and rinse thoroughly with cold water.
2. Return drained chickpeas to saucepan and add 3 cups (750 mL) cold fresh water. Cover and bring to a boil over medium-high heat. Reduce heat and simmer until chickpeas are tender, about 1 hour. Scoop out about 1 cup (250 mL) of the cooking water and set aside. Drain and rinse chickpeas.

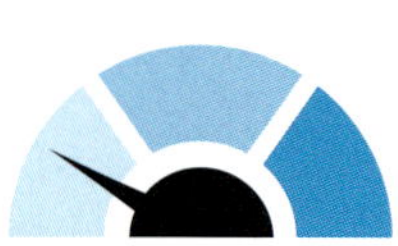
PROTEIN

FIBER

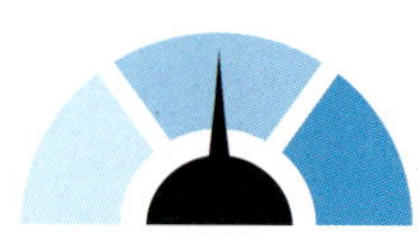
SKILL

**NUTRIENTS PER SERVING**

| | | | | | |
|---|---|---|---|---|---|
| Calories | 127 kcal | Sodium | 161 mg | Vitamin D | 0 mcg |
| Fat | 9 g | Carbohydrate | 10 g | Calcium | 20 mg |
| Saturated fat | 1 g | Fiber | 2 g | Iron | 1 mg |
| Cholesterol | 0 mg | Protein | 4 g | Potassium | 137 mg |

3. In a food processor fitted with metal blade, process cooked chickpeas, tahini, olive oil, ¼ cup (60 mL) of the cooking water and ¼ cup (60 mL) lemon juice until smooth, about 30 seconds, stopping and scraping down sides of the bowl as necessary. If necessary, add additional cooking water and pulse to blend. (You want the mixture to be quite creamy.) Add parsley, 2 cloves garlic, cumin, 1 tsp (5 mL) salt, pepper, and cayenne, if using, and process until smooth, about 15 seconds. Taste and adjust garlic, lemon juice and/or salt to suit your taste. Process again, if necessary. Spoon into a serving bowl and dust with paprika, if using.

## TIPS

If you're in a hurry, instead of setting the chickpeas aside to soak, cover the pot and bring to a boil. Boil for 3 minutes. Turn off heat and soak for 1 hour. Drain and rinse thoroughly with cold water. Then proceed with cooking as in Step 2.

For added flavor, when in Step 2, to the water, add garlic, bay leaves or a bouquet garni made from your favorite herbs tied together in a cheesecloth bag.

# Tuna-Filled Cucumber Boats

- LOW CARBOHYDRATE
- MEDITERRANEAN DIET

**MAKES 3 SERVINGS**

**SERVING SIZE: 2 PIECES**

The tuna salad mixture without the cucumber boats is a great dysphagia-friendly snack! Instead of spreading the mixture onto the cucumber boats, scoop the tuna salad from the bowl using the cucumber for a more tremor-friendly approach.

| | | |
|---|---|---|
| 3 | medium cucumbers, ends trimmed and sliced lengthwise | 3 |
| 3 tbsp | light mayonnaise | 45 mL |
| 3 tbsp | plain nonfat Greek yogurt | 45 mL |
| 2 tsp | Dijon mustard | 10 mL |
| 1 tsp | freshly squeezed lemon juice | 5 mL |
| 2 tsp | chopped fresh parsley | 10 mL |
| 1/4 tsp | salt | 1 mL |
| 1/8 tsp | ground black pepper | 0.5 mL |
| 2 | cans (each 5 oz/142 g) water-packed chunk light tuna, drained | 2 |
| 1/2 | medium red onion, finely chopped | 1/2 |
| 1 | stalk celery, finely chopped | 1 |
| 6 | cherry tomatoes, halved lengthwise | 6 |

1. Using a spoon, scrape the seeds out of the cucumbers, leaving a 1-inch (2.5 cm) canal. Cut the cucumbers in half and place on a plate or cutting board.
2. In a medium bowl, combine the mayonnaise, Greek yogurt, mustard, lemon juice, parsley, salt and pepper. Add the tuna, onion and celery; stir to combine.
3. Spread the tuna mixture evenly in the canal of each cucumber piece. Top each with 1 tomato half. Serve immediately or store in an airtight container in the refrigerator for up to 4 days.

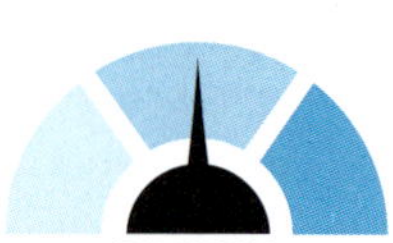
PROTEIN

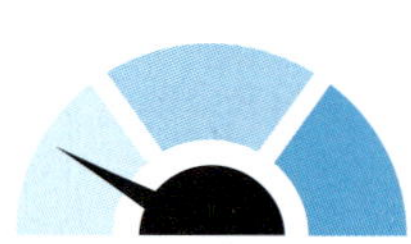
FIBER

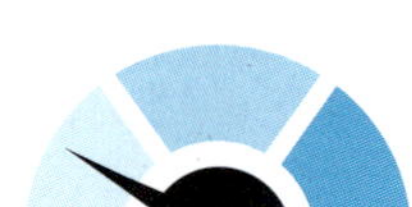
SKILL

**NUTRIENTS PER SERVING**

| | | | | | |
|---|---|---|---|---|---|
| Calories | 139 kcal | Sodium | 530 mg | Vitamin D | 1 mcg |
| Fat | 4 g | Carbohydrate | 13 g | Calcium | 72 mg |
| Saturated fat | 1 g | Fiber | 2 g | Iron | 2 mg |
| Cholesterol | 21 mg | Protein | 13 g | Potassium | 558 mg |

# Smoked Salmon Crostini

- HIGH CALORIE
- MEDITERRANEAN DIET

**MAKES 6 SERVINGS**

**SERVING SIZE: 4 PIECES**

The combination of salmon and olive oil makes this snack an anti-inflammatory powerhouse for brain health.

### TIPS

English cucumbers work well in appetizers like these because they have fewer seeds and are less watery than the regular slicer cucumbers typically found at grocery stores. For very thin slices of cucumber, use a mandoline slicer.

To minimize food waste, dip leftover cucumber slices in extra cream cheese mixture, hummus or your dressing of choice.

- Preheat the oven to 400°F (200°C)

| | | |
|---|---|---|
| ¾ | baguette, preferably whole wheat | ¾ |
| 3 tbsp | olive oil | 45 mL |
| ¾ cup | whipped cream cheese | 175 mL |
| 2 tbsp | chopped fresh dill | 30 mL |
| ⅛ tsp | ground black pepper | 0.5 mL |
| ¾ | English cucumber, thinly sliced (48 slices) | ¾ |
| 4 oz | smoked salmon, cut into 24 bite-size pieces | 125 g |
| 3 tbsp | capers | 45 mL |

1. Cut the baguette on a diagonal into twenty-four ¼-inch (0.5 cm) slices. Arrange them in an even layer on a baking sheet.
2. Brush the olive oil over both sides of the baguette slices. Bake, turning the slices over halfway through, until the bread is golden brown, about 8 minutes.
3. In a small bowl, combine the cream cheese, dill and black pepper, and mix well.
4. To assemble, spread about 1 tsp (5 mL) of the cream cheese mixture over each toasted baguette slice. Press 2 cucumber slices on the top of the cream cheese mixture and then place 1 piece of smoked salmon over the cucumbers. Garnish each with 2 or 3 capers.

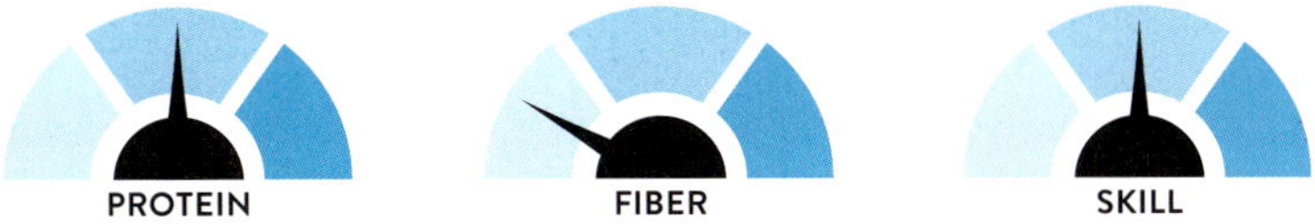


**NUTRIENTS PER SERVING**

| | | | | | |
|---|---|---|---|---|---|
| Calories | 360 kcal | Sodium | 766 mg | Vitamin D | 194 mcg |
| Fat | 24 g | Carbohydrate | 27 g | Calcium | 100 mg |
| Saturated fat | 8 g | Fiber | 0 g | Iron | 1 mg |
| Cholesterol | 37 mg | Protein | 12 g | Potassium | 206 mg |

# Sweet Potato Rounds with Goat Cheese, Pecans and Cranberries

**MAKES 6 SERVINGS**

**SERVING SIZE: 3 ROUNDS**

This recipe pairs antioxidant-rich sweet potatoes and cranberries with protein and healthy fats to create a flavorful appetizer or snack.

- Preheat the oven to 425°F (220°C)
- Baking sheet, coated with nonstick cooking spray

| | | |
|---|---|---|
| 2 | sweet potatoes, sliced into eighteen ½-inch (1 cm) rounds (see Tips, opposite) | 2 |
| 2 tbsp | olive oil | 30 mL |
| ¼ tsp | kosher salt | 1 mL |
| ⅛ tsp | ground black pepper | 0.5 mL |
| ½ cup | raw pecans, coarsely chopped | 125 mL |
| 4 oz | chèvre (fresh goat cheese) | 125 g |
| 1 tbsp | pure maple syrup | 15 mL |
| ¼ tsp | dried thyme | 1 mL |
| ½ cup | dried cranberries | 125 mL |

1. In a large bowl, place the sweet potato rounds. Add the oil, salt and pepper. Toss to evenly coat the potatoes.
2. Place the sweet potato rounds in a single layer about ½ inch (1 cm) apart on the prepared baking sheet. Bake until slightly browned, 22 to 25 minutes, flipping halfway through. Let the sweet potatoes cool for at least 10 minutes. Use a spatula to transfer the rounds to a serving plate.
3. While the sweet potatoes are in the oven, heat the pecans in a small skillet over medium-low heat, stirring occasionally, until slightly toasted, about 5 minutes. Transfer the toasted pecans to a clean bowl.

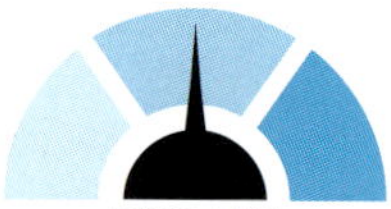
PROTEIN

FIBER

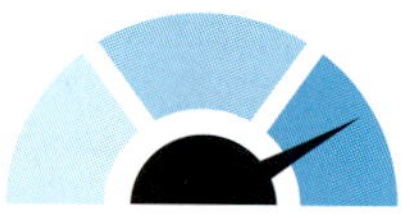
SKILL

**NUTRIENTS PER SERVING**

| | | | | | |
|---|---|---|---|---|---|
| Calories | 291 kcal | Sodium | 134 mg | Vitamin D | 0 mcg |
| Fat | 16 g | Carbohydrate | 32 g | Calcium | 277 mg |
| Saturated fat | 4 g | Fiber | 3 g | Iron | 1 mg |
| Cholesterol | 13 mg | Protein | 7 g | Potassium | 12 mg |

### TIPS

Use long, narrow sweet potatoes for even rounds. Be sure to thoroughly dry them after washing to allow them to brown.

Swap the cranberries for raisins, tart cherries or small pieces of dried fruit of your choice.

4. In a medium bowl, use the back of a fork to mash the goat cheese. Add the maple syrup and thyme and stir to combine.

5. On each round, spoon about 1 tsp (5 mL) of the cheese mixture and, using a butter knife, spread across the top of the sweet potato round. Top with about 1 tsp (5 mL) of the pecans and 1 tsp (5 mL) of the cranberries. Using clean fingers, gently push down on the toppings so they stick to the cheese mixture. Serve immediately.

# Sugar and Spice Nuts

- HIGH-CALORIE
- MEDITERRANEAN DIET
- MIND DIET

**MAKES 1 SERVING**

This recipe elevates a simple handful of nuts, which are a source of protein, healthy fats and fiber. Walnuts specifically are a great source of omega-3 fatty acids, which are essential for protecting brain cells.

## TIPS

An equal amount of roasted seeds (sunflower seeds, green pumpkin seeds) can be used in place of the nuts.

- 12- to 16-oz (375 to 500 mL) mug
- Foil-covered plate, sprayed with nonstick cooking spray

| | | |
|---|---|---|
| 1 tbsp | packed brown sugar | 15 mL |
| 1⁄8 tsp | pumpkin pie spice | 0.5 mL |
| 1⁄2 tsp | water | 2 mL |
| 1⁄3 cup | roasted salted mixed nuts | 75 mL |

1. In the mug, combine brown sugar, pumpkin pie spice and water until blended. Stir in nuts until coated.
2. Microwave on High for 45 seconds. Stir. Checking at 1 minute, then every 10 seconds, microwave on High for 1 to 2 minutes or until syrup begins to harden. Pour onto prepared plate, separating nuts with a fork. Let cool completely.

### CINNAMON SUGAR NUTS

Replace the brown sugar with granulated sugar and replace the pumpkin pie spice with ground cinnamon.

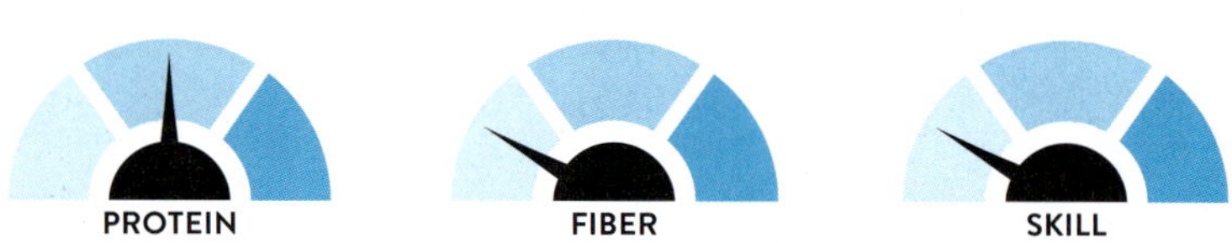


**NUTRIENTS PER SERVING**

| | | | | | |
|---|---|---|---|---|---|
| Calories | 324 kcal | Sodium | 76 mg | Vitamin D | 0 mcg |
| Fat | 24 g | Carbohydrate | 23 g | Calcium | 65 mg |
| Saturated fat | 3 g | Fiber | 3 g | Iron | 1 mg |
| Cholesterol | 0 mg | Protein | 9 g | Potassium | 302 mg |

# Strawberry Kiwi Almond Yogurt Bark

- MEDITERRANEAN DIET
- MIND DIET

**MAKES 6 SERVINGS**

**SERVING SIZE: 4 PIECES**

This recipe is so versatile! Change it up by choosing your favorite flavor of nonfat Greek yogurt, various types of nuts and a combination of fruits. A balanced finger food snack to satisfy the sweet tooth of those with difficulty using utensils.

### TIP

Swap the almonds for pistachios, peanuts, cashews or even sunflower seeds.

- Rimmed baking sheet, lined with parchment paper

| | | |
|---|---|---|
| 2 cups | vanilla-flavored nonfat Greek yogurt | 500 mL |
| | Zest of 1 orange | |
| 8 | strawberries, diced | 8 |
| 2 | kiwifruit, peeled and diced | 2 |
| ½ cup | unsalted dry roasted almonds, coarsely chopped | 125 mL |

1. In a medium bowl, add the yogurt and stir in half of the orange zest. Spoon the yogurt mixture onto the prepared baking sheet and use a spatula to spread it evenly to the edges. It should be about ½ inch (1 cm) thick.
2. Evenly sprinkle the yogurt with the strawberries, kiwis and almonds, and then dust the remaining zest over the yogurt.
3. Place the baking sheet in the freezer for at least 4 hours or until the yogurt sets. Gently break the yogurt bark into 24 pieces. Store in a sealable container in the freezer for up to 2 weeks.

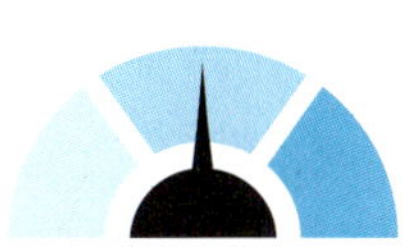
PROTEIN

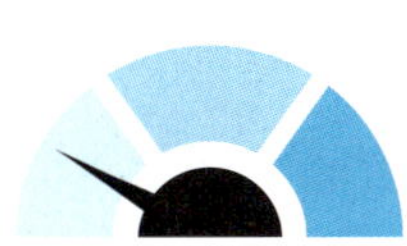
FIBER

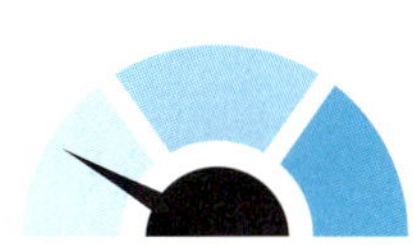
SKILL

**NUTRIENTS PER SERVING**

| | | | | | |
|---|---|---|---|---|---|
| Calories | 135 kcal | Sodium | 27 mg | Vitamin D | 0 mcg |
| Fat | 6 g | Carbohydrate | 13 g | Calcium | 100 mg |
| Saturated fat | 1 g | Fiber | 3 g | Iron | 1 mg |
| Cholesterol | 6 mg | Protein | 10 g | Potassium | 206 mg |

# Greek Yogurt Peanut Butter Dip

- DYSPHAGIA-FRIENDLY
- HIGH-CALORIE

**MAKES 1 SERVING**

This is a great high-calorie, high-protein snack for people that need help gaining weight. Banana slices are a great choice for a dysphagia-friendly option.

## TIPS

For best results, be sure to use Greek yogurt (which is very thick and creamy), not regular plain yogurt.

Any other creamy nut or seed butter (almond, cashew, sesame) can be used in place of the peanut butter.

- 12- to 16-oz (375 to 500 mL) mug

| | | |
|---|---|---|
| 1 tbsp | packed brown sugar or liquid honey | 15 mL |
| 1 tbsp | creamy peanut butter | 15 mL |
| ¾ cup | plain Greek yogurt | 175 mL |
| ¼ tsp | vanilla extract | 1 mL |
| ⅛ tsp | ground cinnamon | 0.5 mL |

***Suggested Accompaniments***

**Apple wedges; grapes; banana slices; pretzel sticks; graham crackers**

1. In the mug, combine brown sugar and peanut butter until smooth. Microwave on High for 15 to 30 seconds or until peanut butter is melted.
2. Stir in yogurt, vanilla and cinnamon until blended and smooth. Serve with any of the suggested accompaniments, as desired.

## PB&J DIP

Omit the cinnamon. Spoon 1 tbsp (15 mL) raspberry preserves on top of the finished dip, then swirl it into the dip with the tip of knife.

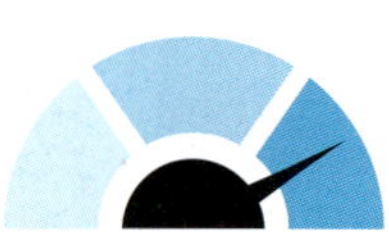
PROTEIN

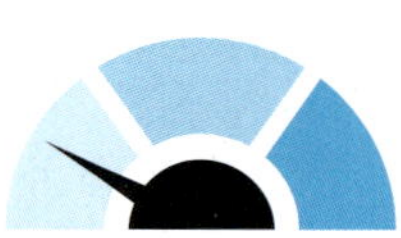
FIBER

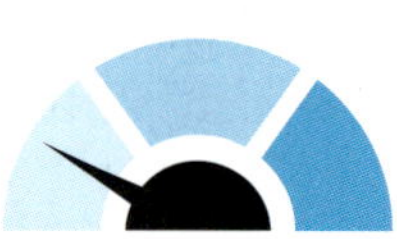
SKILL

**NUTRIENTS PER SERVING**

| | | | | | |
|---|---|---|---|---|---|
| Calories | 384 kcal | Sodium | 155 mg | Vitamin D | 75 mcg |
| Fat | 25 g | Carbohydrate | 27 g | Calcium | 323 mg |
| Saturated fat | 12 g | Fiber | 0 g | Iron | 1 mg |
| Cholesterol | 56 mg | Protein | 16 g | Potassium | 111 mg |

# Chocolate Strawberry Chia Pudding

- DYSPHAGIA-FRIENDLY
- HIGH CALORIE
- MEDITERRANEAN DIET
- MIND DIET

**MAKES 2 SERVINGS**

**SERVING SIZE: ABOUT ½ CUP (125 ML)**

This could be served as a snack, breakfast or dessert! Chia seeds absorb liquid, making them soft and easy to swallow. They travel through the GI tract to help manage constipation. This is a must-try for a quick high-fiber snack.

## TIPS

To lighten up the pudding, use reduced-fat or low-fat chocolate milk.

To make the dish dairy-free, use your favorite plant-based chocolate milk, such as soy milk or almond milk.

- Two 8-oz (250 mL) glass jars with lids

| | | |
|---|---|---|
| 1 cup | chocolate milk | 250 mL |
| ¼ cup | chia seeds | 60 mL |
| 4 | strawberries, quartered | 4 |

1. Pour ½ cup (125 mL) of the chocolate milk in each jar. Add 2 tbsp (30 mL) of the chia seeds to each jar and stir to combine.
2. Divide the strawberries evenly between the jars.
3. Cover each jar and refrigerate overnight.

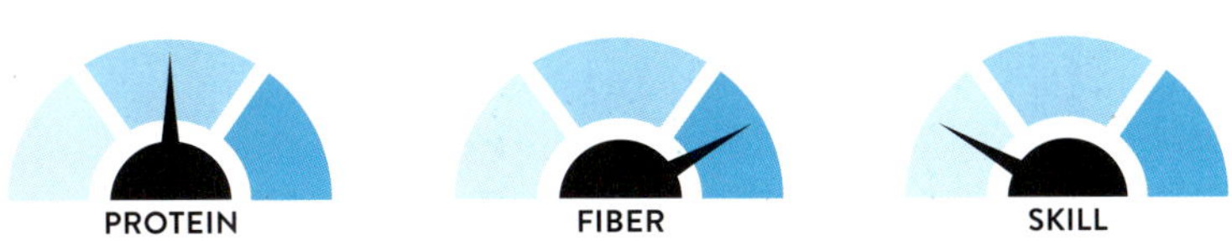


**NUTRIENTS PER SERVING**

| | | | | | |
|---|---|---|---|---|---|
| Calories | 330 kcal | Sodium | 170 mg | Vitamin D | 1 mcg |
| Fat | 11 g | Carbohydrate | 53 g | Calcium | 341 mg |
| Saturated fat | 1.5 g | Fiber | 15 g | Iron | 3 mg |
| Cholesterol | 5 mg | Protein | 11 g | Potassium | 396 mg |

# Cashew Date Bars with Chocolate Drizzle

- MEDITERRANEAN DIET
- MIND DIET

**MAKES 8 SERVINGS**

**SERVING SIZE: 1 BAR**

Simple ingredients for a delicious and convenient snack! Dates are a great source of fiber, and cashews provide protein and healthy fats. Make these ahead of time to take for an after-workout snack or an extra boost of energy when going to doctor's appointments.

- 8-inch (20 cm) square glass baking dish, lined with parchment paper
- Blender or food processor

| | | |
|---|---|---|
| 1 cup | raw cashews, coarsely chopped | 250 mL |
| 1½ cups | pitted dates | 375 mL |
| 2 oz | 60% bittersweet (dark) chocolate (see Tip, opposite) | 60 g |
| ⅛ tsp | salt | 0.5 mL |

1. In a small skillet over medium-low heat, toast the cashews until slightly browned, 3 to 4 minutes. Remove from the heat and let cool for at least 10 minutes.
2. Add the cooled cashews, dates and salt to a blender or food processor. Pulse, scraping down the sides with a wooden spoon occasionally, until the batter is a smooth paste.
3. Spoon the batter into the prepared baking dish (or divide between two dishes, if using) and, using clean fingers, push it into the baking dish and even out the top. Cover and refrigerate until the bars solidify, at least 15 minutes and up to 24 hours.
4. Place the chocolate in a microwave-safe bowl and heat on High, stirring every 20 seconds, until melted, about 1 minute.

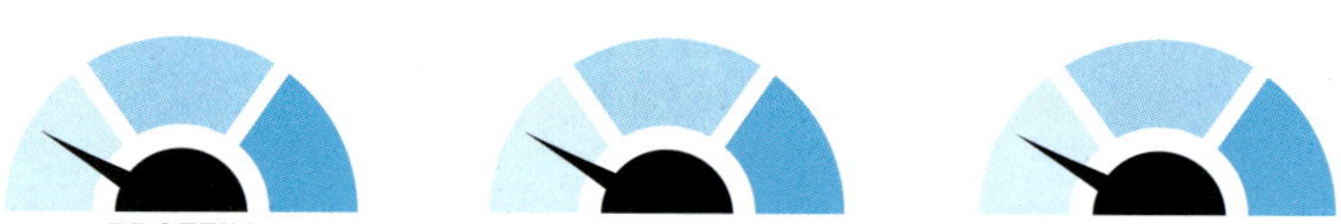

PROTEIN FIBER SKILL

**NUTRIENTS PER SERVING**

| | | | | | |
|---|---|---|---|---|---|
| Calories | 200 kcal | Sodium | 40 mg | Vitamin D | 0 mcg |
| Fat | 9 g | Carbohydrate | 30 g | Calcium | 25 mg |
| Saturated fat | 2.5 g | Fiber | 3 g | Iron | 2 mg |
| Cholesterol | 0 g | Protein | 4 g | Potassium | 197 mg |

**TIP**
Swap the dark chocolate for white chocolate, milk chocolate or semisweet chocolate.

5. Remove the baking dish from the refrigerator and use a spoon to drizzle the chocolate over the bars. Place the baking dish back into the refrigerator to set the chocolate, at least 2 hours.

6. Carefully remove the bars by pulling out the parchment paper and place on a cutting board. Using a sharp knife or pizza cutter, cut into eight even bars and serve. Store leftovers in a sealable container in the refrigerator for up to 5 days.

# Fruit Bars

- MEDITERRANEAN DIET
- MIND DIET

**MAKES 6 BARS**

**SERVING SIZE: 1 BAR**

A small snack with a good amount of fiber! Drizzle with melted peanut butter for even more calories and protein to support muscle maintenance. For people with forgetfulness, having snacks like these within sight can be helpful reminders to eat throughout the day.

**TIP**
Store the bars in an airtight container in the refrigerator for up to 2 weeks.

- Food processor or blender
- 9- by 5-inch (23 by 12.5 cm) metal loaf pan, lined with parchment paper

| | | |
|---|---|---|
| 1 cup | almond flour | 250 mL |
| 1 cup | mixed dried fruit (such as blueberries, cherries and cranberries) | 250 mL |
| ½ cup | roughly chopped pitted dates | 125 mL |
| Pinch | salt | Pinch |

1. In a food processor or blender, combine the almond flour, dried fruit, dates and a pinch of salt. Pulse in 5-second intervals, scraping down the sides of the container as necessary, until the mixture becomes pliable. Gradually increase the interval time until you can process continuously and the mixture forms a ball (the timing will depend on the strength of the machine).
2. Scrape the mixture into the prepared pan and press it flat.
3. Place plastic wrap directly on the surface and refrigerate until set, at least 1 hour or overnight. Remove from the pan, using the parchment liner. Remove the plastic wrap, then cut into bars. Eat cold or at room temperature.

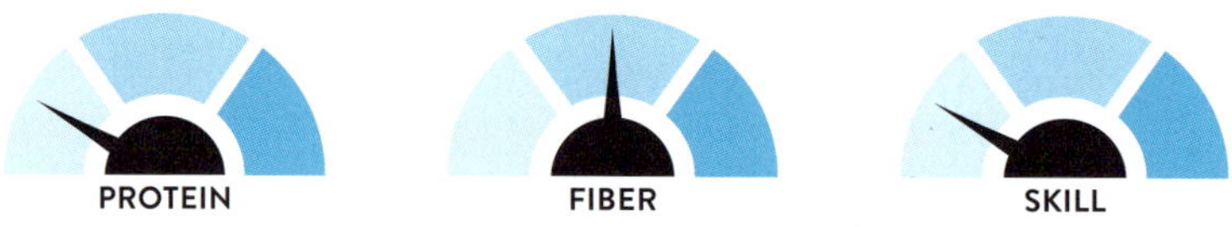


**NUTRIENTS PER SERVING**

| | | | | | |
|---|---|---|---|---|---|
| Calories | 198 kcal | Sodium | 7 mg | Vitamin D | 0 mcg |
| Fat | 8 g | Carbohydrate | 30 g | Calcium | 57 mg |
| Saturated fat | 1 g | Fiber | 4 g | Iron | 1 mg |
| Cholesterol | 0 mg | Protein | 4 g | Potassium | 326 mg |

# Tropical Green Smoothie

- DYSPHAGIA-FRIENDLY
- MEDITERRANEAN DIET
- MIND DIET

**MAKES 2 SERVINGS**

**SERVING SIZE: 1½ CUPS (375 ML)**

While the coconut milk adds a tropical flair, you can substitute for a low-fat cow's milk for a lower-fat version of this refreshing beverage. For more protein, try substituting the coconut milk for an over-the-counter protein shake or add your favorite protein powder!

**TIP**

Swap the spinach for chopped kale.

- Blender

| | | |
|---|---|---|
| 1 cup | lightly packed baby spinach | 250 mL |
| ¾ cup | frozen mango chunks | 175 mL |
| ¾ cup | frozen pineapple chunks | 175 mL |
| 1 | medium banana, halved | 1 |
| 1 cup | unsweetened light coconut milk | 250 mL |

1. In a blender, combine the spinach, mango, pineapple, banana and coconut milk; blend on high speed until smooth, about 1 minute.
2. Divide evenly between two glasses and serve immediately.

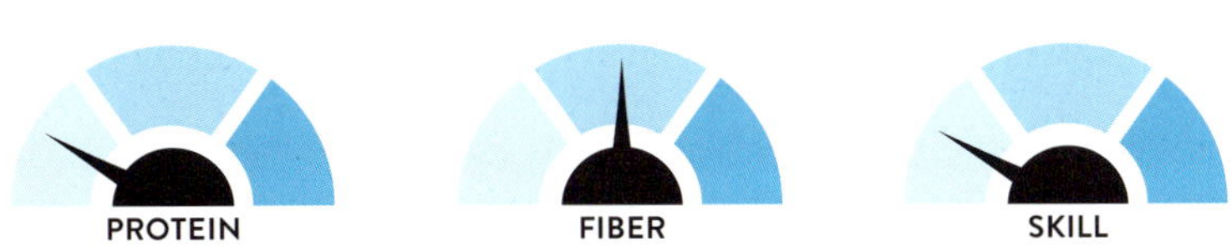


**NUTRIENTS PER SERVING**

| | | | | | |
|---|---|---|---|---|---|
| Calories | 140 kcal | Sodium | 12 mg | Vitamin D | 2 mcg |
| Fat | 3 g | Carbohydrate | 31 g | Calcium | 79 mg |
| Saturated fat | 2 g | Fiber | 4 g | Iron | 1 g |
| Cholesterol | 0 mg | Protein | 2 g | Potassium | 457 mg |

# Pumpkin Pie Smoothie

**DYSPHAGIA-FRIENDLY**

**MAKES 2 SERVINGS**

**SERVING SIZE: 1 CUP (250 ML)**

For a high-calorie smoothie, choose whole milk and/or full-fat Greek yogurt. For a higher-protein version, use more Greek yogurt or add your choice of protein powder.

### TIP

If you want to give your smoothie a little more kick, add an additional ¼ tsp (1 mL) pumpkin pie spice.

- Blender

| | | |
|---|---|---|
| 1 | medium banana, halved | 1 |
| ¾ cup | canned 100% pumpkin | 175 mL |
| ¾ cup | vanilla nonfat Greek yogurt | 175 mL |
| ¾ cup | nonfat milk | 175 mL |
| 2 tbsp | roughly chopped raw walnuts | 30 mL |
| ¾ tsp | pumpkin pie spice | 3 mL |

1. In a blender, combine the banana, pumpkin purée, Greek yogurt, milk, walnuts and pumpkin pie spice; blend on high speed until smooth, about 1 minute.
2. Divide evenly between two glasses and serve immediately.

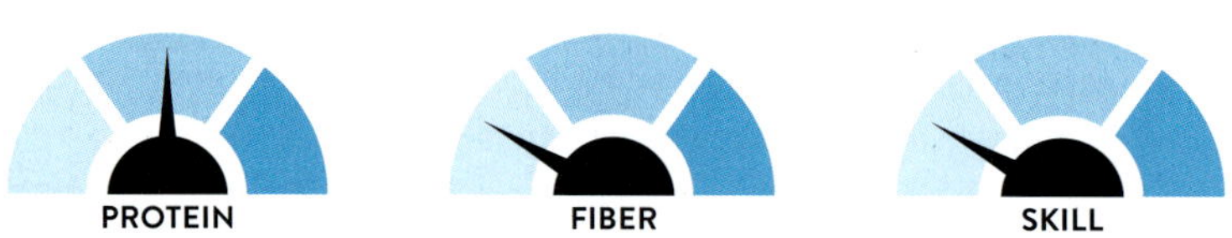


**NUTRIENTS PER SERVING**

| | | | | | |
|---|---|---|---|---|---|
| Calories | 229 kcal | Sodium | 70 mg | Vitamin D | 1 mcg |
| Fat | 5 g | Carbohydrate | 35 g | Calcium | 246 mg |
| Saturated fat | 1 g | Fiber | 6 g | Iron | 2 mg |
| Cholesterol | 8 mg | Protein | 13 g | Potassium | 504 mg |

# Strawberry Kiwi Smoothie

DYSPHAGIA-FRIENDLY

**MAKES 2 CUPS (500 ML)**

**SERVING SIZE: 1 CUP (250 ML)**

This smoothie is full of fruit and a good amount of fiber, which could help relieve constipation if consumed as part of a balanced diet.

### TIPS

To extract the flesh from kiwifruit, use a paring knife to remove a small amount of skin from the bottom. Carefully insert a small spoon between the flesh and the skin and rotate it until the skin becomes loose. Scoop out the flesh.

For a creamy smoothie, substitute an equal amount of almond milk for the orange juice and add 3 tbsp (45 mL) melted coconut oil.

- Blender

| | | |
|---|---|---|
| 1 cup | freshly squeezed orange juice | 250 mL |
| 2 | kiwifruit, peel removed | 2 |
| 1 | banana, halved | 1 |
| 8 to 10 | strawberries | 8 to 10 |
| 1 tsp | raw agave nectar | 5 mL |
| 1 tsp | alcohol-free organic vanilla extract | 5 mL |

1. In blender, combine orange juice, kiwis, banana, strawberries, agave nectar and vanilla. Blend at high speed until smooth. Serve immediately.

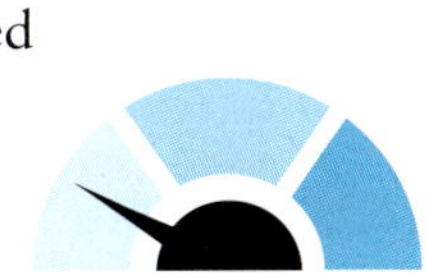
PROTEIN

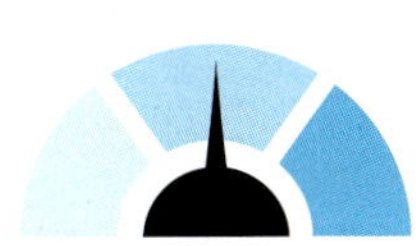
FIBER

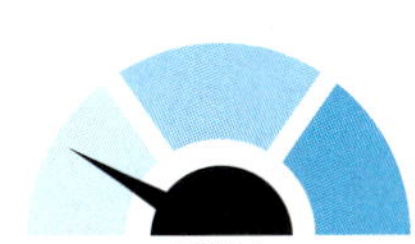
SKILL

**NUTRIENTS PER SERVING**

| | | | | | |
|---|---|---|---|---|---|
| Calories | 210 kcal | Sodium | 5 mg | Vitamin D | 0 mcg |
| Fat | 1 g | Carbohydrate | 50 g | Calcium | 71 mg |
| Saturated fat | 0 g | Fiber | 7 g | Iron | 1 mg |
| Cholesterol | 0 mg | Protein | 3 g | Potassium | 819 mg |

CHAPTER 15

# DESSERTS

# Chocolate Trail Mix Bark

▸ HIGH-CALORIE

**MAKES 1 SERVING**

This is a great dessert to satisfy your sweet tooth and boost your fiber intake!

**TIP**

Substitute vegetable oil or coconut oil instead of the butter if desired.

- 12- to 16-oz (375 to 500 mL) mug
- Small plate, lined with waxed paper or parchment paper

| | | |
|---|---|---|
| 2 tbsp | semisweet chocolate chips | 30 mL |
| ½ tsp | butter | 2 mL |
| ¼ cup | coarsely chopped assorted raw, toasted or roasted nuts | 60 mL |
| 2 tbsp | raw or roasted sunflower seeds | 30 mL |
| 2 tbsp | chopped dried fruit (such as apricots, cranberries or raisins) | 30 mL |
| 1 tbsp | flaked or shredded unsweetened coconut | 15 mL |

1. In the mug, microwave chocolate chips and butter on High for 30 seconds. Stir. Microwave in 10-second intervals, stopping to stir after each, until chocolate is melted and mixture is smooth.
2. Stir in nuts, seeds, dried fruit and coconut until well coated. Scoop mixture onto prepared plate, spreading slightly with back of spoon. Freeze for 10 to 15 minutes or until set. Break into bite-size pieces.

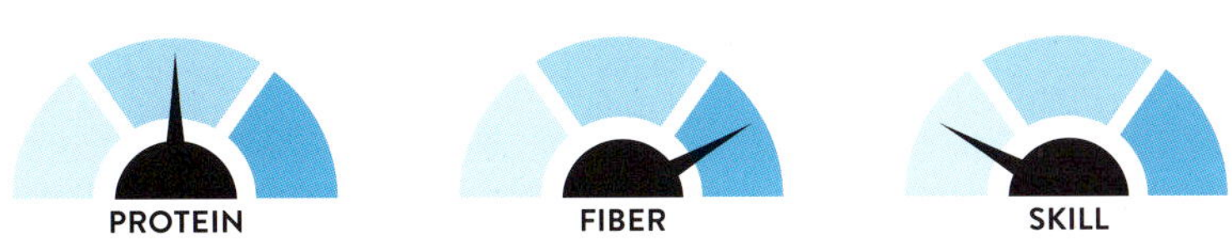


**NUTRIENTS PER SERVING**

| | | | | | |
|---|---|---|---|---|---|
| Calories | 526 kcal | Sodium | 12 mg | Vitamin D | 0 mcg |
| Fat | 40 g | Carbohydrate | 40 g | Calcium | 58 mg |
| Saturated fat | 13 g | Fiber | 8 g | Iron | 3 mg |
| Cholesterol | 5 mg | Protein | 12 g | Potassium | 518 mg |

# High-Protein Chocolate Mug Muffin

▸ DYSPHAGIA-FRIENDLY

**MAKES 1 SERVING**

A high-protein dessert for people on a protein redistribution diet or high-protein diet. The banana makes for a moist muffin with added fiber and flavor.

## TIPS

If you have a choice, opt for an all-natural protein powder (stevia-sweetened, no artificial colors or flavors). They are increasingly available in the health food sections of grocery stores.

You can use 2 tbsp (30 mL) beaten egg in place of the egg white.

- 16-oz (500 mL) mug, sprayed with nonstick cooking spray

| | | |
|---|---|---|
| ¼ cup | chocolate whey protein powder | 60 mL |
| 1½ tsp | unsweetened cocoa powder | 7 mL |
| ¼ tsp | baking powder | 1 mL |
| Pinch | salt | Pinch |
| 1 | large egg white | 1 |
| ½ cup | mashed very ripe banana | 125 mL |
| 1 tbsp | milk | 15 mL |

1. In the mug, combine protein powder, cocoa powder, baking powder and salt. Using a fork, beat in egg white, banana and milk until very well blended.
2. Microwave on High for 1 to 2 minutes (checking at 1) or until center is just set. Let cool slightly or entirely in mug. Eat directly from mug or gently serve on plate.

### BANANA VANILLA PROTEIN MUFFIN

Use vanilla whey protein powder in place of the chocolate and omit the cocoa powder.

### PUMPKIN SPICE PROTEIN MUFFIN

Use vanilla whey protein powder in place of the chocolate and omit the cocoa powder. Replace the banana with ¼ cup (60 mL) unsweetened pumpkin purée (not pie filling) and increase the milk to ¼ cup (60 mL). Add ¼ tsp (1 mL) pumpkin pie spice or ground cinnamon and 1 packet (about ¼ tsp/1 mL) of powdered stevia or stevia-blend sweetener with the baking powder.

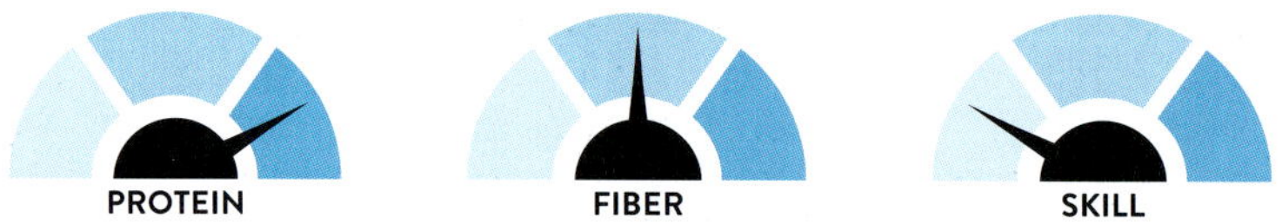


**NUTRIENTS PER SERVING**

| | | | | | |
|---|---|---|---|---|---|
| Calories | 212 kcal | Sodium | 321 mg | Vitamin D | 0 mcg |
| Fat | 2 g | Carbohydrate | 31 g | Calcium | 330 mg |
| Saturated fat | 1 g | Fiber | 4 g | Iron | 1 mg |
| Cholesterol | 16 mg | Protein | 21 g | Potassium | 519 mg |

# Silky Chocolate Mousse

- DYSPHAGIA-FRIENDLY
- HIGH CALORIE
- MEDITERRANEAN DIET

**MAKES 4 SERVINGS**

The incorporation of plant-based protein and limited added sugar ingredients makes this a balanced Mediterranean-style dessert. Substitute tofu for avocado for an even higher-calorie version of this dysphagia-friendly dessert option.

### TIP

Cacao powder is powdered raw chocolate. It is similar to cocoa powder but tastes even better, with a deeper, richer flavor. Cacao powder is available in well-stocked supermarkets and natural food stores and online. You may substitute an equal quantity of good-quality cocoa powder.

- Food processor

| | | |
|---|---|---|
| 1 | block (12 oz/375 g) medium-firm silken tofu | 1 |
| 1 cup | raw cacao powder (see Tip, left) | 250 mL |
| $^3/_4$ cup | raw agave nectar | 175 mL |
| $^1/_2$ tsp | alcohol-free organic vanilla extract | 2 mL |

1. In food processor fitted with the metal blade, combine tofu, cacao powder, agave nectar and vanilla. Process until smooth, stopping the motor to scrape down sides of work bowl as necessary.
2. Transfer to a serving bowl. Serve immediately or cover and refrigerate for up to 5 days.

### CHOCOLATE AVOCADO MOUSSE

Substitute 2 ripe avocados for the tofu.

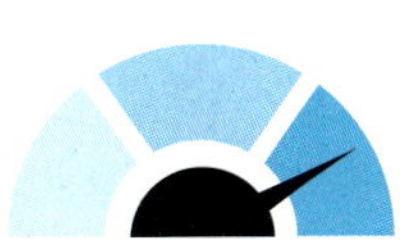


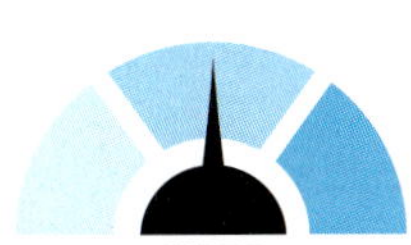


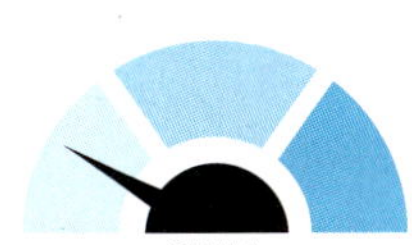


**NUTRIENTS PER SERVING**

| | | | | | |
|---|---|---|---|---|---|
| Calories | 330 kcal | Sodium | 25 mg | Vitamin D | 0 mcg |
| Fat | 4 g | Carbohydrate | 63 g | Calcium | 279 mg |
| Saturated fat | 0 g | Fiber | 7 g | Iron | 8 mg |
| Cholesterol | 0 mg | Protein | 15 g | Potassium | 349 mg |

# Chewy Oatmeal Coconut Cookies with Cranberries and Pecans

- LOW CARBOHYDRATE
- MEDITERRANEAN DIET
- MIND DIET

**MAKES ABOUT 48 COOKIES**

**SERVING SIZE: 1 COOKIE**

Using whole wheat flour and rolled oats adds complex carbohydrates to this yummy dessert. This means there's more fiber and sustained energy than if you were to use refined grains. The cranberries, nuts and coconut give these cookies flavor and antioxidants. Desserts are allowed in moderation on the MIND and Mediterranean diets. It's all about balance.

- Preheat oven to 350°F (180°C)
- Baking sheets, lightly greased or lined with parchment paper

| | | |
|---|---|---|
| ¾ cup | whole wheat pastry flour | 175 mL |
| ¾ cup | whole barley flour | 175 mL |
| 1 tsp | baking powder | 5 mL |
| ½ tsp | salt | 2 mL |
| 1 cup | butter, softened | 250 mL |
| 1 cup | packed Demerara or other raw cane sugar | 250 mL |
| 1 | egg | 1 |
| 1 tsp | vanilla extract | 5 mL |
| ½ cup | liquid honey | 125 mL |
| 2 cups | old-fashioned (large-flake) rolled oats | 500 mL |
| 1 cup | sweetened flaked coconut | 250 mL |
| ½ cup | dried cranberries | 125 mL |
| ½ cup | chopped pecans | 125 mL |

1. In a bowl, combine whole wheat and barley flours, baking powder and salt.
2. In a large bowl, beat using handheld electric mixer, butter and sugar until light and creamy. Add egg, vanilla and honey, beating and scraping down the sides of the bowl until blended. Gradually add flour mixture, beating until smooth. Stir in oats, coconut, cranberries and pecans.

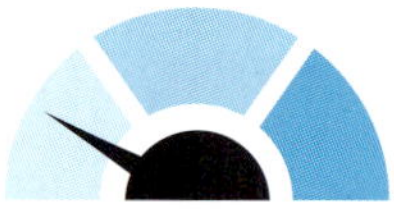
PROTEIN

FIBER

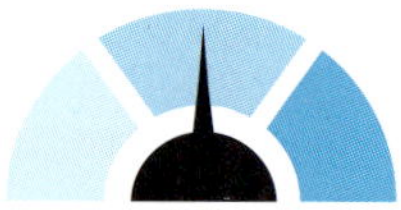
SKILL

**NUTRIENTS PER SERVING**

| | | | | | |
|---|---|---|---|---|---|
| Calories | 107 kcal | Sodium | 40 mg | Vitamin D | 0 mcg |
| Fat | 5 g | Carbohydrate | 16 g | Calcium | 26 mg |
| Saturated fat | 1 g | Fiber | 2 g | Iron | 0 mg |
| Cholesterol | 4 mg | Protein | 2 g | Potassium | 63 mg |

3. Drop dough by tablespoonfuls (15 mL), about 2 inches (5 cm) apart, on prepared baking sheets. Bake in preheated oven until golden, about 12 minutes. Let cool for 5 minutes on sheets, then transfer to a wire rack and let cool completely.

### TIPS

These cookies are a bit soft when they come out of the oven, but they firm up while cooling. Make sure they are just golden while baking—they continue to cook on the sheet after removal from the oven.

If you don't like nuts, eliminate the pecans and double the quantity of cranberries. Similarly, if you don't like cranberries, leave them out and double the amount of pecans.

# Gingerbread Chia Pudding

- DYSPHAGIA-FRIENDLY
- HIGH CALORIE
- MEDITERRANEAN DIET

**MAKES 4 SERVINGS**

**SERVING SIZE: 1 JAR**

This could serve as a dessert or a sweet breakfast item that is convenient to make the night before! Chia seeds pack in lots of fiber to support gut health.

**TIP**

Want even more flavor? Add sliced bananas and a drizzle of maple syrup before serving!

- Four 4-oz (125 mL) jars with lids

| | | |
|---|---|---|
| 2 tbsp | pure maple syrup | 30 mL |
| 2 tsp | unsulfured molasses | 10 mL |
| 1 tsp | vanilla extract | 5 mL |
| 1 tsp | ground cinnamon | 5 mL |
| ¼ tsp | grated fresh gingerroot | 1 mL |
| ¼ tsp | ground nutmeg | 1 mL |
| ¼ tsp | ground allspice | 1 mL |
| ⅛ tsp | salt | 0.5 mL |
| 2 cups | unsweetened almond milk or nonfat milk | 500 mL |
| ½ cup | chia seeds | 125 mL |
| ¼ cup | raw or unsalted roasted chopped pecans | 60 mL |
| ¼ cup | dark chocolate chips | 60 mL |

1. In a medium bowl, whisk together the maple syrup, molasses, vanilla, cinnamon, ginger, nutmeg, allspice and salt. Slowly whisk in the almond milk until incorporated.
2. Pour about ½ cup (125 mL) of the almond milk mixture into each of the glass jars. Add 2 tbsp (30 mL) of the chia seeds into each jar and stir until well combined. Cover the jars and refrigerate for at least 8 hours and up to 24 hours.
3. To serve, open the jars and top each with 1 tbsp (15 mL) of the pecans and 1 tbsp (15 mL) of the dark chocolate chips. Serve immediately.

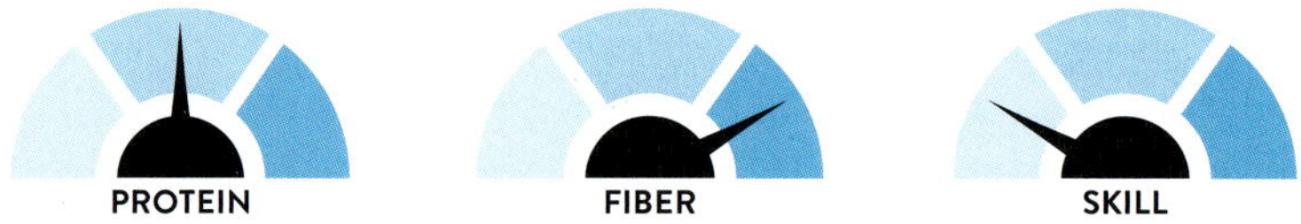


**NUTRIENTS PER SERVING**

| | | | | | |
|---|---|---|---|---|---|
| Calories | 324 kcal | Sodium | 258 mg | Vitamin D | 55 mcg |
| Fat | 22 g | Carbohydrate | 32 g | Calcium | 456 mg |
| Saturated fat | 5 g | Fiber | 14 g | Iron | 3 mg |
| Cholesterol | 0 mg | Protein | 9 g | Potassium | 254 mg |

# Brie and Blueberry Bundles

- KETOGENIC DIET
- LOW CARBOHYDRATE

**MAKES 8 PASTRIES**

**SERVING SIZE:**
**1 PASTRY**

This savory, sweet dessert takes little effort but packs lots of flavor! Pair with fresh blueberries or strawberries to add fiber, vitamins and minerals.

## TIPS

You can use any jam or jelly you like. For a spicy twist, try hot red pepper jelly.

Store the bundles in an airtight container in the refrigerator for up to 3 days.

Rewarm these bundles for 10 to 15 minutes on the middle rack of an oven preheated to 250°F (120°C). Do not microwave.

- Preheat the oven to 375°F (190°C)
- 12-cup muffin pan

| | | |
|---|---|---|
| 2 | sheets puff pastry dough, each 10 inches (25 cm) square, thawed if frozen (1 lb/500 g) | 2 |
| 3 oz | Brie cheese, cut into eight ½-inch (1 cm) cubes | 90 g |
| 3 tbsp | blueberry jam | 45 mL |

1. Place one sheet of dough on a lightly floured work surface. Using a sharp knife or pizza cutter, cut the sheet into four 5-inch (12.5 cm) squares.
2. Place a pastry square over one well of the muffin pan. Place a Brie cube in the center and press lightly to push the pastry into the well without breaking it. Place 1 tsp (5 mL) blueberry jam directly on top of the Brie. Fold the corners of the pastry into the center over the filling. Pinch the edges together where they touch to form four seams.
3. Repeat steps 1 and 2 with the second sheet of dough, the remaining Brie and the remaining jam. You will have 8 bundles.
4. Bake in the preheated oven until the pastry is a deep golden all over, about 20 to 25 minutes.
5. Let cool in the pan on a wire rack for 5 minutes before removing. Eat warm.

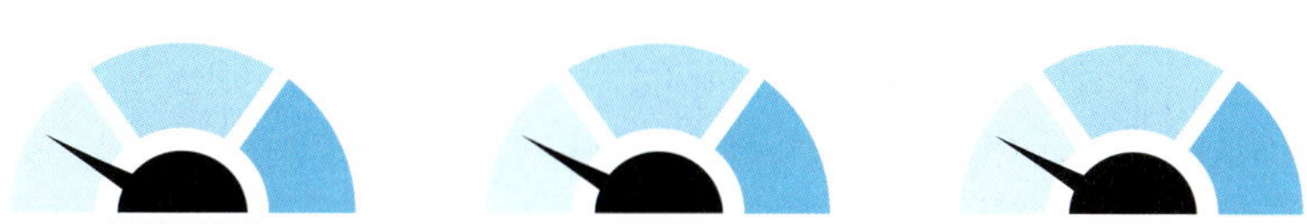


**NUTRIENTS PER SERVING**

| | | | | | |
|---|---|---|---|---|---|
| Calories | 155 kcal | Sodium | 177 mg | Vitamin D | 4 mcg |
| Fat | 9 g | Carbohydrate | 14 g | Calcium | 23 mg |
| Saturated fat | 5 g | Fiber | 0 g | Iron | 1 mg |
| Cholesterol | 7 mg | Protein | 1 g | Potassium | 46 mg |

# Lemon Pots

- DYSPHAGIA-FRIENDLY
- HIGH CALORIE

**MAKES 6 SERVINGS**

**SERVING SIZE: ½ CUP (125 ML) RAMEKIN**

This citrus dessert is high-calorie for those looking to maintain or gain weight, and it is easier to swallow for those with swallowing difficulty. With simple steps, it can be made in no time for those looking to effortlessly satisfy their sweet tooth.

### TIP

Leftover lemon pots (without the whipped cream topping) can be covered and stored in the refrigerator for up to 5 days.

- Six ½-cup (125 mL) ramekins, glasses or mason jars
- Electric mixer

| | | |
|---|---|---|
| 2 | lemons | 2 |
| 2½ cups | heavy or whipping (35%) cream, divided | 625 mL |
| ⅔ cup | granulated sugar | 150 mL |

1. Grate the zest from the lemons and juice them, making 2 tbsp (30 mL) zest and ½ cup (125 mL) juice. (Reserve any extra for another use.)
2. In a small saucepan, whisk together 2 cups (500 mL) cream, the sugar, 1 tbsp (15 mL) lemon zest and the lemon juice. Bring to a boil over medium heat, then reduce to a simmer and cook for 3 minutes, stirring constantly. Remove from the heat and let cool for 15 minutes.
3. Pour an equal quantity of the mixture into each ramekin. Cover and refrigerate until set, at least 6 hours, or overnight. Set aside the remaining 1 tbsp (15 mL) lemon zest in an airtight container for garnishing later.
4. In a small bowl, using an electric mixer on high speed, whip the remaining cream until stiff peaks form. Top the lemon pots with a dollop of whipped cream and a sprinkle of lemon zest before serving.

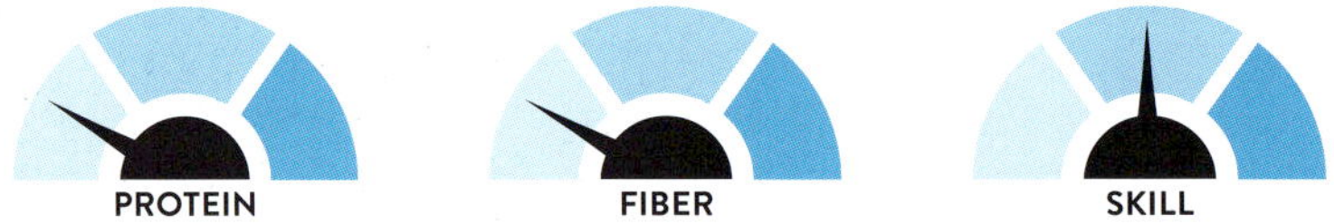


**NUTRIENTS PER SERVING**

| | | | | | |
|---|---|---|---|---|---|
| Calories | 425 kcal | Sodium | 27 mg | Vitamin D | 63 mcg |
| Fat | 36 g | Carbohydrate | 26 g | Calcium | 70 mg |
| Saturated fat | 23 g | Fiber | 0 g | Iron | 0 mg |
| Cholesterol | 113 mg | Protein | 3 g | Potassium | 131 mg |

# Frozen Pecan and Caramel Log

**MAKES ABOUT 16 TO 20 COOKIES**

**SERVING SIZE: 1 COOKIE**

A classic chocolate, caramel and nuts combination, this sweet treat can be made in bulk in advance. Enlist the help of your family or friends to make the caramel if heating elements are tricky for you.

### TIP

When adding the cream to the caramel there is quite a bit of steam that is released, so be sure to not have your face or arms over the pan to avoid severe burns.

| | | |
|---|---|---|
| 2 oz | bittersweet chocolate, coarsely chopped | 60 g |
| 2 cups | coarsely chopped toasted pecans | 500 mL |
| 1 cup | granulated sugar | 250 mL |
| ¼ cup | water | 60 mL |
| ⅓ cup | heavy or whipping (35%) cream | 75 mL |

1. In a heatproof bowl, stir together chocolate and pecans. Set aside.
2. In a saucepan, combine sugar and water. Heat over medium heat, stirring gently, just until sugar is dissolved, then bring to a boil, without stirring. Boil gently (reducing heat if necessary), without stirring, until syrup turns a caramel color. Remove from heat and let bubbles subside. Carefully pour in cream (see Tip, left) and swirl to incorporate.
3. Immediately pour caramel over the nuts and chocolate and stir to coat. Place a 12-inch (30 cm) square of parchment paper on a work surface. Pour the nut mixture over the paper. Starting with the edge closest to you, using the parchment to lift the nut mixture as you would a sushi rolling mat, roll up to form a log about 2 inches (5 cm) in diameter and 8 to 10 inches (20 to 25 cm) long. Place the wrapped log on a square of plastic wrap and wrap up tightly, twisting both ends to make the log as tight as possible. Freeze for at least 3 hours, until firm, or for up to 2 weeks.
4. Remove from plastic wrap and place log (leaving the paper on) on a cutting board. Cut into ½-inch (1 cm) thick cookies, remove the paper and serve immediately.

PROTEIN

FIBER

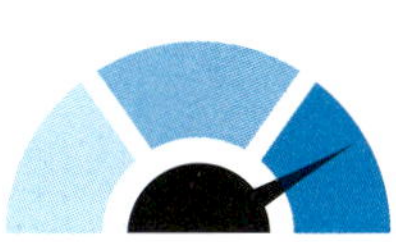
SKILL

**NUTRIENTS PER SERVING**

| | | | | | |
|---|---|---|---|---|---|
| Calories | 153 kcal | Sodium | 1 mg | Vitamin D | 0 mcg |
| Fat | 11 g | Carbohydrate | 14 g | Calcium | 13 mg |
| Saturated fat | 3 g | Fiber | 1 g | Iron | 0 mg |
| Cholesterol | 5 mg | Protein | 1 g | Potassium | 73 mg |

# Cranberry Pear Brown Betty

**MAKES 7 SERVINGS**

With minimal ingredients and simple steps, this dessert is one that can be made ahead and be ready just in time for an after-dinner sweet treat. This is a more balanced dessert as it uses whole wheat flour and fruits with minimal added sugars.

## TIPS

To make dry bread crumbs for this recipe, toast 4 slices of whole wheat bread. Tear into pieces and process in a food processor fitted with a metal blade until finely ground.

Use a light whole wheat loaf. Those with a heavy molasses content will overpower the fruit.

If you don't have stevia, use ¼ cup (60 mL) brown sugar (such as Demerara) or evaporated cane juice sugar (such as Sucanat).

- Works best in a small (3½-quart) slow cooker
- Greased slow cooker stoneware

| | | |
|---|---|---|
| **2 cups** | **dry whole wheat bread crumbs (see Tips, left)** | **500 mL** |
| **2 tbsp** | **butter, melted, or extra-virgin olive oil** | **30 mL** |
| **6** | **pears, peeled, cored and sliced** | **6** |
| **1 cup** | **fresh or frozen cranberries** | **250 mL** |
| **2 tbsp** | **stevia extract (see Tips, left)** | **30 mL** |
| **1 tbsp** | **freshly squeezed lemon juice** | **15 mL** |
| **½ cup** | **cranberry juice** | **125 mL** |

1. In a bowl, combine bread crumbs and butter. Set aside.
2. In a large bowl, combine pears, cranberries, stevia and lemon juice.
3. Spread one-third of the bread crumb mixture in prepared stoneware. Layer half the pear mixture over top. Repeat. Finish with remaining crumbs mixture and pour cranberry juice over top. Cover and cook on High for 4 hours, until fruit is tender and mixture is hot and bubbly.

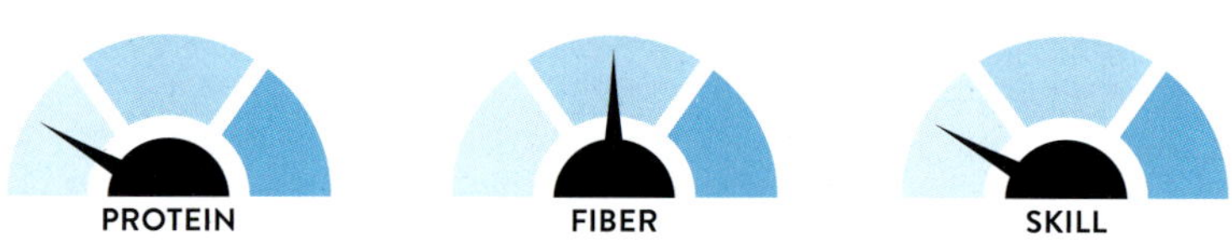


**NUTRIENTS PER SERVING**

| | | | | | |
|---|---|---|---|---|---|
| Calories | 251 kcal | Sodium | 124 mg | Vitamin D | 0 mcg |
| Fat | 4 g | Carbohydrate | 49 g | Calcium | 14 mg |
| Saturated fat | 1 g | Fiber | 6 g | Iron | 1 mg |
| Cholesterol | 0 mg | Protein | 3 g | Potassium | 200 mg |

# Apple Blackberry Crisp

- MEDITERRANEAN DIET
- MIND DIET

**MAKES 5 SERVINGS**

Adding rolled oats to this tasty dessert increases the fiber content to help support gut health. This dessert highlights key recommendations of both the MIND and Mediterranean diets — berries and whole grains.

## TIPS

Some apples are better for eating and some are better for baking. The best baking apples are ones that hold their shape when cooked, such as Cortland, Honeycrisp and Granny Smith.

Cover the casserole dish or transfer leftovers to an airtight container and store in the fridge for up to 3 days.

- **Preheat the oven to 350°F (180°C)**
- **6-cup (1.5 L) casserole dish, greased**

| | | |
|---|---|---|
| **3 cups** | **peeled and diced baking apples (about 3 large; see Tips, left)** | **750 mL** |
| **1 cup** | **fresh blackberries** | **250 mL** |
| **1⁄3 cup** | **lightly packed brown sugar, divided** | **75 mL** |
| **1 tbsp** | **freshly squeezed lemon juice** | **15 mL** |
| **2 tsp** | **ground cinnamon** | **10 mL** |
| **1 1⁄4 cups** | **large-flake (old-fashioned) rolled oats** | **310 mL** |
| **1⁄3 cup** | **vegan butter** | **75 mL** |
| | **Vegan vanilla ice cream (optional)** | |

1. To a large bowl, add the apples, blackberries, 1 tbsp (15 mL) brown sugar, lemon juice and cinnamon; stir gently to coat. Pour into the prepared casserole dish, reserving the bowl. Set aside.
2. In the reserved bowl, combine the oats and remaining 1⁄4 cup (60 mL) brown sugar. Using two knives or a pastry blender, cut the vegan butter into the oats mixture until crumbly.
3. Spread the oats topping evenly over the fruit mixture. Bake in the preheated oven for 35 to 40 minutes, until the top is golden brown.
4. Let cool for 5 to 10 minutes. Serve warm with a scoop of vegan vanilla ice cream on top (if using).

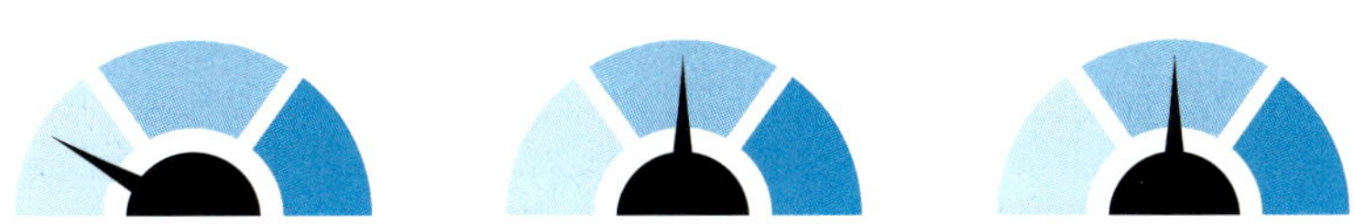


**NUTRIENTS PER SERVING**

| | | | | | |
|---|---|---|---|---|---|
| Calories | 283 kcal | Sodium | 81 mg | Vitamin D | 0 mcg |
| Fat | 12 g | Carbohydrate | 42 g | Calcium | 54 mg |
| Saturated fat | 10 g | Fiber | 6 g | Iron | 1 mg |
| Cholesterol | 4 mg | Protein | 4 g | Potassium | 218 mg |

# Mom's Super-Moist Banana Loaf

- DYSPHAGIA-FRIENDLY
- LOW CARBOHYDRATE
- MEDITERRANEAN DIET
- MIND DIET

**MAKES 2 LOAVES, 12 SLICES EACH**

**SERVING SIZE: 1 SLICE**

The use of bananas and applesauce in this recipe not only adds moisture but also adds fiber! Choose a whole-grain flour and substitute vegetable oil with extra-virgin olive oil for a more Mediterranean-forward approach. Freeze the leftover loaf for a quick dessert later.

- Preheat oven to 350°F (180°C)
- Two 9- by 5-inch (23 by 12.5 cm) metal loaf pans, greased

| | | |
|---|---|---|
| $2\frac{1}{2}$ cups | whole wheat flour | 625 mL |
| $1\frac{1}{2}$ tsp | ground cinnamon | 7 mL |
| $1\frac{1}{4}$ tsp | baking powder | 6 mL |
| $1\frac{1}{4}$ tsp | baking soda | 6 mL |
| 1 tsp | ground nutmeg | 5 mL |
| $\frac{1}{2}$ tsp | salt | 2 mL |
| $\frac{1}{4}$ tsp | ground cloves | 1 mL |
| $\frac{1}{2}$ cup | granulated sugar | 125 mL |
| 2 | eggs | 2 |
| $\frac{2}{3}$ cup | buttermilk | 150 mL |
| 2 tbsp | vegetable oil | 30 mL |
| $1\frac{1}{2}$ cups | mashed ripe bananas | 375 mL |
| $\frac{2}{3}$ cup | unsweetened applesauce | 150 mL |

1. In a large bowl, combine flour, cinnamon, baking powder, baking soda, nutmeg, salt and cloves.
2. In a medium bowl, whisk together sugar, eggs, buttermilk and oil until blended. Stir in bananas and applesauce. Pour over flour mixture and stir until just combined.
3. Pour batter into prepared loaf pans, dividing equally. Bake in preheated oven for 40 to 45 minutes or until a tester inserted in the center comes out clean. Let cool in pans on a wire rack for 10 minutes, then transfer to rack to cool completely.

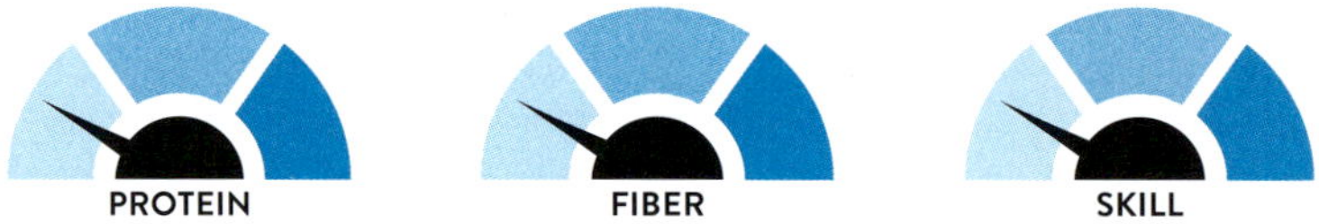


**NUTRIENTS PER SERVING**

| | | | | | |
|---|---|---|---|---|---|
| Calories | 93 kcal | Sodium | 130 mg | Vitamin D | 0 mcg |
| Fat | 2 g | Carbohydrate | 18 g | Calcium | 49 mg |
| Saturated fat | 0 g | Fiber | 2 g | Iron | 0 mg |
| Cholesterol | 16 mg | Protein | 3 g | Potassium | 118 mg |

## Acknowledgments

We sincerely thank Dr. Jeanette Andrade and students Courtney Sroka, Michelle Loew, Rachel Stennett, Muna Aboushaar, Avery Little and Mary Kim for their support and contributions to the nutrition analysis of the recipes in this book. Their time and effort are greatly appreciated.

# Contributing Authors

Toby Amidor
*The Best Rotisserie Chicken Cookbook: Over 100 Tasty Recipes Using a Store-Bought Bird*
Recipes from this book are found on pages 167 and 198.

Toby Amidor
*The Best 3-Ingredient Cookbook: 100 Fast and Easy Recipes for Everyone*
Recipes from this book are found on pages 228, 239 and 240.

Toby Amidor
*The Family Immunity Cookbook: 101 Easy Recipes to Boost Health*
Recipes from this book are found on pages 140, 144, 156, 159, 193, 200, 204, 219, 220, 223 and 238.

Toby Amidor
*Up Your Veggies: Flexitarian Recipes for the Whole Family*
Recipes from this book are found on pages 147, 158, 164, 166, 218, 229 and 230.

Olivia Biermann
*Liv B's Easy Everyday: 100 Sheet-Pan, One-Pot and 5-Ingredient Vegan Recipes*
Recipes from this book are found on pages 148, 184, 243.

Charmian Christie
*The 3-Ingredient Baking Book: 101 Simple, Sweet and Stress-Free Recipes*
Recipes from this book are found on pages 132, 135, 142, 143, 153, 173, 180, 226 and 238.

Tiffany Collins
*300 Best Casserole Recipes*
Recipes from this book are found on pages 145, 150, 152, 187 and 196.

Judith Finlayson
*Sensational Slow Cooker Gourmet*
Recipes from this book are found on pages 208 and 242.

Judith Finlayson
*The Complete Whole Grains Cookbook: 150 Recipes for Healthy Living*
Recipes from this book are found on pages 134, 182, 202 and 236.

Judith Finlayson and Jordan Wagman
*750 Best Appetizers: From Dips & Salsas to Spreads & Shooters*
Recipes from this book are found on pages 215, 216 and 241.

Douglas McNish
*Vegan Everyday: 500 Plant-Based Recipes*
Recipes from this book are found on pages 136, 162, 174, 178, 231 and 235.

Emily Richards and Sylvia Kong
*Best of Bridge Kitchen Simple: 125 Quick and Easy Recipes*
Recipes from this book are found on pages 138, 160, 168, 170, 172, 177, 181 and 192.

Emily Richards and Sylvia Kong
*Best of Bridge Done in One: Perfect Recipes in One Pot, Pan or Skillet*
Recipes from this book are found on pages 131, 146, 155, 163, 194, 195, 206, 210, 211 and 213.

Camilla V. Saulsbury
*250 Best Meals in a Mug: Delicious Homemade Microwave Meals in Minutes*
Recipes from this book are found on pages 133, 190, 222, 224, 233 and 234.

Karrie Truman
*Seriously Good Freezer Meals: 150 Easy Recipes to Save Your Time, Money & Sanity*
Recipes from this book are found on pages 137, 169 and 191.

Mary Sue Waisman
Dieticians of Canada
*Cook! 275 Recipes Celebrate Food from Field to Table*
Recipes from this book are found on pages 171, 186, 188, 197, 214 and 244.

# Index

# C

# D

## I



## J



## K



## L



## M

## N



## O



## P

## Q

# R



# S

## T



## U



## V



## W

# X



# Y



# Z



**Library and Archives Canada Cataloguing in Publication**

Title: The Parkinson's plate : a health & diet guide to manage your journey / Dr. Michael S. Okun, MD & Emily Truscott, MS, RD, LD.
Names: Okun, Michael S., author. | Truscott, Emily. author.
Description: Includes index.
Identifiers: Canadiana 20260172847 | ISBN 9780778807414 (softcover)
Subjects: LCSH: Parkinson's disease—Diet therapy—Popular works. | LCSH: Parkinson's disease—Patients—Nutrition—Popular works. | LCSH: Parkinson's disease—Diet therapy—Recipes. | LCSH: Parkinson's disease—Popular works. | LCGFT: Cookbooks.
Classification: LCC RC382 .O39 2026 | DDC 616.8/330654—dc23